HEAL

YOUR

WHOLE
BODY

HEAL
YOUR
WHOLE
BODY

The **12-DAY POWER PLAN**
to Flush Toxins, Balance Hormones
& Reset Your Body's
Most Essential Organ

FRANCES MURCHISON, HHC, AADP

RODALE.

To Jay, my rock

© 2014 by Frances Murchison

Exercise photographs © 2014 by Rodale Inc.

Illustrations © 2014 by Jay Sidebotham

Printed in the United States of America
Rodale Inc. makes every effort to use acid-free ∞, recycled paper ♻.

Candid photographs were supplied by the individuals participating in the LiverUp! Cleanse.

Exercise photographs by Thomas MacDonald/Rodale Images
Book design by Elizabeth Neal

Library of Congress Cataloging-in-Publication Data is on file with the publisher.

ISBN 978–1–62336–037–5 direct hardcover

6 8 10 9 7 5   Direct mail hardcover

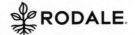

We inspire and enable people to improve their lives and the world around them.
For more of our products, visit rodalestore.com or call 800–848–4735.

CONTENTS

ACKNOWLEDGMENTS

So many people have helped make this book a reality. I want to thank them for their special role in this project—and for their presence in my life.

- To the hundreds of cleansers who've dared to take on the Liver Up! cleanse with me. They have taught me about courage, patience, and radical acceptance.

- To Nancy Fitzgerald, my wonderful editor, who suggested I write a book on the amazing benefits of the Liver Up! cleanse.

- To my beloved husband, Jay, who told me to say "Yes." Following his dharma, he's taught me so much about grace, gratitude, and perseverance.

- To my beautiful children, John Reid and Helen, who bring joy and light into my life.

- To my cherished Poppy, who told me I could accomplish anything to which I put my heart and mind and who may be the oldest Liver Up! cleanser. At 85, he's hugely energetic, strong, and open-hearted—living proof that cleansing works.

- To my dear friend Deborah, who has taught me most of what I know about food, yoga, and life on life's terms. Her honest voice, open mind, and compassionate heart inspire me to live into mine.

- To my friend, colleague, and yoga instructor Jess for her smile and encouragement.

- To my friend Bill, who saved the day when my hard drive died.

- To my dear friends Vanessa and Darby, whose generosity enabled me to complete this book.

- And, finally, to all the folks at Rodale who are committed to improving the health and lives of their readers. It is a privilege to be among their contributors.

FOREWORD

Heal Your Whole Body is an important book that's filled with medical information about all that your wonderful liver does, plus much-needed guidance for improving your health. It's good to have a book that focuses on your liver, which is an amazing factory for nutrition, biochemistry, and detoxification.

I often say that detoxification is the missing link in Western nutrition. It provides a break from some of our daily habits. In this book, Frances Murchison thoroughly explains the importance of detoxifying your body and mind, and gives details on toxins to avoid and nutrients to include for best long-term health.

The detox process offers so many benefits. I just finished my 3-week autumn detox group at my office last night, and the results were amazing. Everyone dropped some weight and felt better, experiencing improved digestion, energy, and sleep, and having more vibrant-looking skin. Some reduced or got off of their blood pressure medicines as their high numbers dropped to normal and stayed there. A participant with type 2 diabetes got his out-of-control blood sugar into a healthier range. But most importantly, everyone exchanged old habits for healthy new ones. Many are drinking high-nutrient brews instead of coffee, and all participants took a break from sugars and alcohol. You can experience an astonishing array of benefits from following a program like the one you'll find in the book in your hands right now.

However, following the program takes some reading and learning, and then some reorganization, especially of your lifestyle. And you know what? You are totally worth it! Often, it's your attitude that needs to be shifted first, and in *Heal Your Whole Body*, Frances puts this change front and center. She is a gifted writer and nutritionist with a unique perspective, and she has experience working with people to make positive changes and improvements to their health. Her wisdom will guide you through making those changes in your own life.

When I did my first cleanse in 1975, my health improved as my weight came down and my allergies cleared up. More importantly, I felt better than I ever had before. I had lots of energy, I slept better, and my congestion disappeared. Mostly, I experienced a wonderful new feeling of life's vitality and potential. I said to myself, "Elson, this is how you want to feel—every day!"

What you put into your body matters. Everything you consume becomes part of you. The basic, most important message you should take away from reading *Heal Your Whole Body* is this: "This is the only body I have, and I am going to treat it with love." When I experienced this attitude shift, I was able to make better choices in what I ate. I was motivated to exercise regularly. I made sure to get quality sleep. I learned to manage my stress and express myself emotionally. I wanted to be the best *me* I could be.

This book can do the same for you. It can empower you if you apply its messages and follow its sage advice. I have reviewed many books on detoxifying the body, and Frances has a very good one here—with all of the guidelines you need to follow and positive, healing ideas and programs. This book will educate you about the qualities of foods and herbs, and you'll see why they should become part of your balanced and energizing diet. And you'll find a beautiful selection of nutritionally rich yet detoxifying recipes to nourish you during this process.

Particularly crucial to your detox process is learning to heal your gut, which is essential to long-term health and vitality. Pay careful attention to Chapter 4. Healthy bacteria (probiotics) are important to know about and utilize as one of the tools in your repertoire of health aids.

Another hugely important aspect of Frances's book is the section on learning how to relax and calm your mind. She'll teach you about yoga, which quiets your spirit and strengthens your body. One of the original maxims of holistic medicine, after all, is to keep your life in balance—

body, mind, heart, and spirit. This is a worthy goal. All of our parts are important, and it's worthwhile to take the time and energy to nourish them all.

So give some of the ideas and practices in *Heal Your Whole Body* a try. Put your health back into your own hands by taking responsibility for the choices you make, and decide to eat in a different way to see and experience your potential for optimal energy and health. You are totally worth it!

—Elson M. Haas, MD
Integrative, Holistic Family Medicine Practitioner
Author of *Staying Healthy with the Seasons, The Detox Diet,* and
Staying Healthy with Nutrition
Sebastopol, California

CHAPTER 1

Liver 101

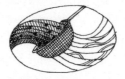

Your liver is your body's powerhouse. It's responsible for many of the processes that keep your body functioning optimally. A healthy liver plays a key role in relieving digestive issues, such as sluggish metabolism, gas, bloating, and constipation. It regulates blood sugar levels, which—when out of balance—cause sugar cravings, fatigue, fuzzy thinking, and hypoglycemia. A toxic liver can lead to inflammatory diseases, such as diabetes, arthritis, atherosclerosis, high blood pressure, and autoimmune diseases, as well as hormonal imbalances that can cause headaches, mood swings, and depression. In addition to these and many more functions, your liver plays an important role in maintaining a healthy weight.

In short, your liver is vital in creating and sustaining equilibrium in your body. Healing, nourishing, and supporting it may be the single most important practice you can pursue to reclaim wholeness in body, mind, and spirit. Caring for such a complex and powerful organ requires great vigilance regarding what you allow into your body. Unfortunately, you may unknowingly be subjecting your liver to injury every day.

With every breath you take, every bite you chew, every drink you swallow, your liver must filter every single item that enters your body. Consider the chemicals you consume regularly—from pollution, pesticides, preservatives, processed foods, and plastics to hormone-laden foods, herbicides, and heavy metals. These toxins overload your liver, compromising its ability to perform its many jobs.

While it's one of the most abused organs in the body, your liver may also be one of the most forgiving. It can lose three-quarters of its cells before it stops functioning, and it's the only organ that can regenerate itself. So when you become proactive about nourishing and supporting your liver, it can respond quickly. When your liver can accomplish its wide variety of jobs, you reap the benefits: increased energy, clearer thinking, fewer food cravings, and more control over your weight.

Clearly, your liver is very important. So how do you help it keep you healthy, balanced, and energized? What can you do when it's not working at its best? That's what this book is all about. You'll learn about the essential role your liver plays in determining your health and well-being—and most important, you'll learn a simple program to help you heal and strengthen your liver and restore your health. Let's get started!

The Basics

What's the largest—and maybe even the most important—organ inside your body? Your heart? Your brain? Your lungs? No. It's your lowly liver— the unglamorous organ we tend to ignore. But that's about to change. Here are some amazing facts: Your 3-pound liver is a maroon-colored miracle of multitasking, carrying out more than 500 jobs. At any given moment, it holds about a pint of blood—that's 13 percent of your body's entire supply. Shaped like a boomerang, it has two large sections—the right and left lobes—that are separated by a fibrous tissue called the falciform ligament. Check out the diagram opposite.

So where does this powerhouse hide? It's sheltered behind your ribs and tucked away in the upper right-hand portion of your abdomen, sitting above your gallbladder and portions of your pancreas and intestines. These organs are all neighbors, working alongside your liver to digest, absorb, and process everything you eat. Here are just a few jobs that your amazing liver performs.

- It serves as your body's primary filtering system.

- It makes and stores fuel, regulating carbohydrate metabolism.

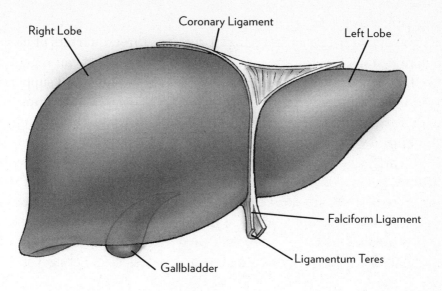

- It manufactures proteins, which transport fats and hormones.

- It produces more than a quart of bile a day, regulating fat metabolism.

- It controls hormonal balances.

Let's take a closer look.

Your Liver Is a Filtering Machine

Know how a pool filter screens out bugs and leaves? Your liver works in much the same way. At an astonishing rate of 3 pints per minute, your liver is the only organ that receives blood from two separate sources: the hepatic vein, which carries oxygen-rich blood from the aorta in your heart, and the portal vein, which carries de-oxygenated blood and digested food from your small intestine. These blood vessels stream into your liver, then subdivide like branches of a tree, terminating in tiny capillaries, each of which leads to a lobule. Thousands of lobules, each

Internal Anatomy of Liver

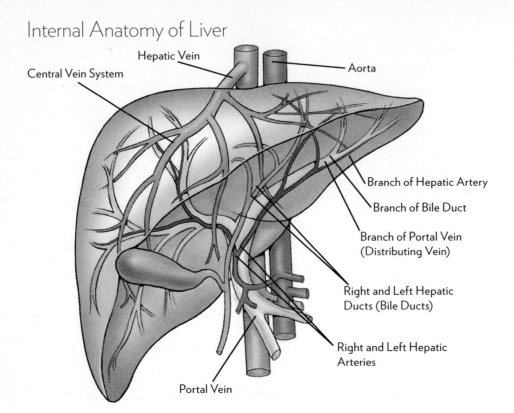

Hepatic Vein

Central Vein System

Aorta

Branch of Hepatic Artery

Branch of Bile Duct

Branch of Portal Vein
(Distributing Vein)

Right and Left Hepatic
Ducts (Bile Ducts)

Right and Left Hepatic
Arteries

Portal Vein

made of hepatic cells, create liver tissue. Within the tissue, over 300 billion specialized cells, connected by a well-organized system of bile ducts and blood vessels that's called the biliary system, make up the liver.

All these cells and ducts work together to filter and transform every single particle that enters your body. Up close and magnified, your liver looks like a giant strainer, designed precisely to remove toxic matter from your bloodstream as it flows through this sieve. It's also very intelligent—it serves as your body's chemical brain and screening station, determining which substances support your body and need to be absorbed and which sabotage your body and need to be filtered out of your bloodstream. The liver is the Einstein of organs: It can recognize millions of potentially harmful external chemicals, known as exotoxins or oxidants, then transform them into something harmless or prepare them for elimination.

And it's always working. Your liver performs its job of filtration every time you drink a cup of coffee or a bottle of beer. Every time you take a bite of food—from luscious, organic, local raspberries to those shipped from Argentina and sprayed with poisonous pesticides—your liver is discerning and filtering what's healing from what's harmful. The liver's filtration job even extends to the toxic elements you breathe and consume in your daily environment, including smog, car exhaust, cigarettes, secondhand smoke, food additives, charred or fried foods, chemicals used in cleaning products, makeup—and even medications and vitamin supplements.

But filtering everything that you consume is just the first part of your liver's job. After that, it must convert those substances to a different form to allow the nutrients and chemical compounds to be:

- Neutralized, as antioxidants counteract free radicals

- Transformed from fat-soluble chemicals into water-soluble ones

- Eliminated from your body through your kidneys, large intestine, and skin

Let's look at exactly what this means.

Cleaning Up a Toxic Wasteland

Your liver is littered with toxins—those that you consume from the outside (exotoxins) and those that your body makes from within (endotoxins). No matter where they originate, it's your liver's job to clean them up or eliminate them. Here's a quick overview.

Exotoxins. There are a few different kinds of toxins that we take in from outside of our bodies—from the foods we eat and the chemicals we're exposed to in our environment.

First, there are oxidants. Regardless of their origin, oxidants are called free radicals, highly reactive chemicals that can cause significant damage to your cells if they're not neutralized properly. Free radicals abound in the standard American diet (SAD). All processed, preserved, pesticide-laden, chemically treated foods contain free radicals. Examples include white flour, margarine, meat from animals raised in confined areas on pesticide-laden feed, partially hydrogenated oils, sugar, and alcohol. When these foods are consumed, your liver comes to the rescue by neutralizing many of these free radicals. In Chapter 2, you'll learn how antioxidants support your liver in neutralizing these toxins.

Many of the toxic chemicals that enter your body are fat (lipid) soluble, which means that they dissolve only in fatty or oily solutions. Lipid-soluble chemicals are attracted to fat tissues and cell membranes, which are made up of fatty substances. And once these toxic chemicals glom on to fat deposits in your body, they can remain there for years, to be released, little by little, during periods of stress, exercise, or fasting. When that happens, you may experience headaches, nausea, fatigue, and dizziness. Examples of fat-soluble toxins are pesticides, heavy metals, preservatives, food additives, pollutants, and plastics.

So how do you get rid of exotoxins? You convert them into water-soluble chemicals. Your liver is designed to do exactly that, through a complex process that involves a system of enzymes. Once this conversion is complete, water-soluble toxins can be excreted from your body via fluids, such as bile, sweat, and urine.

If your liver becomes overloaded, these toxic chemicals tend to accumulate in fatty tissues and organs, such as your brain and hormonal glands (also known as the endocrine system). When that happens, trouble follows, from brain dysfunction to hormonal imbalances such as menstrual disturbances, adrenal gland exhaustion, and early menopause. And to make matters worse, many of these fat-soluble chemicals are carcinogenic—they've been associated with the rising incidence of some cancers.

Endotoxins. Not all of the toxins in your body make their way in from the outside. Some of them are home-grown. Besides filtering and transforming every external compound you consume, your liver filters and cleans your blood of internally created toxins, or endotoxins. Those are natural by-products of body processes. Two examples are ammonia and urea.

Ammonia is a natural by-product of protein digestion. Bacteria living in your digestive tract break down proteins for your body to assimilate and use to repair and grow cells. As protein breaks down, any excess your body can't use is converted to ammonia and is released in your intestine. Your bloodstream absorbs this ammonia and takes it first to your liver. There, through chemical reactions, your liver converts the ammonia into a less-toxic chemical, *urea*, which passes into your kidneys to be released from your body via urine. If your liver is damaged and the cells can't remove ammonia from your blood, the ammonia stays in your blood and enters general circulation—and that spells trouble. It can affect your brain and cause symptoms such as difficulty concentrating, fatigue, irritability, and confusion. Excess ammonia can also damage your nervous system, liver, and kidneys.

So whether it's exotoxins or endotoxins, it's always your liver to the rescue. Your liver filters, transforms, and breaks them all down, then excretes the by-products into bile or blood. Bile by-products enter your intestine and ultimately leave your body in the form of feces. Blood by-products, on the other hand, are filtered out by your kidneys and skin, exiting your body in the form of urine and sweat. If your liver and your body's detoxification pathways are clean and strong, your body can maintain homeostasis—a balanced state of health and wellness.

Dealing with Toxic Overload

If your liver or your body's detoxification pathways become overloaded, all of those toxins accumulate in your blood system, fat cells, and liver. But if they stay too long, your immune system kicks into overdrive, treating these chemicals as if they were invading organisms. Your immune system produces excessive inflammatory chemicals.

Your body produces antibodies when it perceives that it's been exposed to an invading organism. But sometimes it produces autoantibodies, protein-based antibodies, manufactured by your immune system, that mistakenly target your body's own tissues. Usually the immune system is able to discriminate between foreign substances and your body's own cells. When your immune system fails to recognize the invading organism as its own, though, it may produce autoantibodies that attack its own cells, tissues, or organs, causing inflammation and damage. In this hyperstimulated state, your immune system can become susceptible to a variety of immune disorders: allergies; inflammatory diseases, such as rheumatoid arthritis, atherosclerosis, and even cancer; chronic fatigue syndrome; or autoimmune diseases, such as celiac disease, Crohn's disease, multiple sclerosis, rheumatoid arthritis, anemia, lupus; and type 1 diabetes.

} The Scary Seven Food Additives to Avoid

1. Coloring agents (blue 1, blue 2, yellow 5, and yellow 6), found in everything from cakes and candies to macaroni and cheese, sports drinks, and even medicines.

2. Olestra (Olean), a fat substitute found in some potato chips. It can deplete your body of important nutrients and cause serious digestive problems.

3. Brominated vegetable oil (BVO), found in citrus-flavored sodas and sports drinks. It's been linked to serious health issues, including autoimmune disease, cancer, hypothyroidism, and hearing loss.

4. Potassium bromate (brominated flour), found in baked goods like breads, rolls, and bagel chips. It's been associated with kidney and nervous system problems.

5. Azodicarbonamide, found in everything from running shoes to frozen foods to bread. It's been linked to asthma.

6. BHA and BHT, found in foods including butter, meat, and beer. It may be linked to some cancers.

7. rBGH and rBST, synthetic hormones found in dairy products. They've been linked to certain cancers, including breast and colon.

Toxic Chemicals Are . . . }

. . . In Your Home

PFCs
(perfluorinated compounds)
Used in:
- Clothing
- Cookware
- Food Containers
- Carpets

BPA
(bisphenol A)
Used in:
- Food Can Linings
- Baby Bottles
- Receipt Paper
- CDs and DVDs

Formaldehyde
Used in:
- Carpeting
- Soaps and Detergents
- Cabinetry
- Glues and Adhesives

Phthalates
Used in:
- Air Fresheners
- Paper
- Vinyl Tile
- Wood Varnishes and Lacquers

PBDEs
(polybrominated diphenyl ethers)
Used in:
- Furniture
- Electrical Equipment
- TVs and Computers

Toluene
Used in:
- Paints
- Flooring Adhesives
- Plumbing Adhesives
- Adhesive Removers

. . . In Your Body

BPA is found in 9 of 10 Americans

PFCs, **PBDEs**, and **phthalates** are in 99% of pregnant women

232 TOXIC CHEMICALS were found in umbilical cord blood from US newborns

. . . Putting Your Health at Risk

FERTILITY PROBLEMS are linked to PFCs, PBDEs, and phthalates

ASTHMA is linked to toluene and formaldehyde

PARKINSON'S DISEASE is linked to trichloroethylene and other chemicals

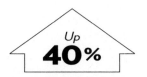

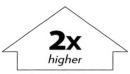

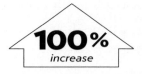

Source: Environmental Defense Fund

Whether it's through toxins in your environment or toxins created in your body, your immune system can suffer. On top of these toxins, we add insult to injury by eating processed and high-carbohydrate foods. But instead of popping pills that suppress the symptoms of immune dysfunction, the most efficient and effective way to cleanse your blood and take the load off of your immune system is to support your hardworking, amazing liver.

Your Liver Is a Fueling Station

Every single moment, your liver is involved in creating, processing, and supplying vast amounts of nutrients that feed up to 100 trillion cells of your body. Each cell produces billions of chemical reactions per second, so to sustain the vast myriad of activities each cell generates, your liver must supply each cell with a constant stream of nutrients, enzymes, and hormones.

To do this, your liver makes glucose—sugar—from the carbohydrates you eat. So when you munch on an apple, your liver transforms the carbs in that piece of fruit into glucose that travels via your blood to the rest of your body, where it's used for energy. If your body can't use all of the glucose at one time, some of it is stored in your liver as glycogen. Then, when your body signals that it needs energy—or when your blood sugar levels are low—your liver comes to the rescue, converting glycogen back into glucose and releasing it into your bloodstream.

But that's not all. If no carbohydrates are available in your body, your liver turns into a carbohydrate factory, manufacturing glucose from both fat and proteins. If your diet is regularly low in carbohydrates, your liver can even convert stored fat into glucose for energy.

Sometimes, though, your diet is loaded with carbs. When that happens, your liver gets overworked and congested with toxic compounds, triggering your immune system and overloading it, potentially causing illness.

Your Liver Is a Protein Machine

Your liver really knows how to work with raw materials. Consider protein: Your liver converts amino acids from protein-based foods like meat or beans into the many different proteins your body needs to perform a variety of functions. These proteins transport fats, hormones, and iron throughout your body. On top of that, your liver produces proteins that regulate fluid balance and immune function. Let's consider a couple of important proteins that the liver keeps in good supply.

High-Density Lipoprotein (HDL). HDL transports cholesterol out of your blood vessel walls to your liver for excretion from your body. Too much cholesterol in your body increases your risk of atherosclerosis, a condition in which fat, cholesterol, and other substances build up on the walls of your arteries and create plaque. Over time, this plaque blocks your arteries and can lead to heart attacks, strokes, and high blood pressure. To keep the right amount of HDL in your bloodstream, your liver needs to be functioning at its optimum.

Albumin. Albumin plays a major role in maintaining fluid balance in your body, creating a gradient in your cells that pulls fluids in when needed and releases fluids when your cells become too full. Your cells are much like water-filled balloons: They can lose fluid and need to be refilled, but if they become too full, they can burst. When albumin levels decrease, water in the plasma of your cells tends to seep into the empty space surrounding the cells where water doesn't usually collect. This fluid leakage can result in swelling in the tissues surrounding the cells.

In addition to regulating fluid movement from your bloodstream to your cells and back, albumin serves as a transport vehicle, moving calcium, the hormone progesterone, and bilirubin (a product that's formed in your liver when red blood cells break down) throughout your tissues. Without sufficient levels of bilirubin, you can experience jaundice, weight loss, and fatigue.

Other Proteins That Your Liver Manufactures. Additional proteins transport waste such as damaged cholesterol, used estrogen, and insulin back to your liver for detoxification and elimination via your kidneys. Your body requires used estrogen to be broken down and excreted daily.

Your Liver Is a Bile Factory

One of your liver's most important functions is to produce bile—up to a quart and a half daily. Bile is a sticky digestive juice that may be yellow, brown, or green. It helps your body with many important tasks.

- It neutralizes gastric fluids.

- It breaks down carbohydrates, fats, and proteins.

- It assimilates fat-soluble vitamins.

- It lubricates your intestines.

- It eliminates drugs, heavy metals, medications, and toxic chemicals from your body.

Bile is an alkaline fluid made up of bile acids (also called bile salts), bilirubin, phospholipids, cholesterol, bicarbonate, and water. Bile salts are made from cholesterol, which either comes from your diet or is made by your liver. They mix with the fats you eat to help your body absorb fats from your intestinal tract. Bilirubin, cholesterol, and phospholipids are end products of metabolism. Bicarbonate, secreted by your stomach, is a major alkaline element in your body, playing a major role in maintaining pH balances. Along with water, it's excreted into your small intestine to help neutralize stomach acid in your intestinal tract. This is important because while protein needs acid enzymes to be digested, carbs and fats need alkaline enzymes for digestion.[1]

The Digestion Connection

Here's a bit of background on what happens when you eat: When you chew and swallow your food, it enters your stomach, where various digestive enzymes, hydrochloric acid, and water break it down to a partially digested semifluid substance called chyme. Depending on what and how much you've eaten, your stomach takes anywhere from 15 minutes to about an hour to convert that meal into chyme.

When chyme moves from your stomach into the first part of your small intestine, the duodenum, it's usually very acidic. To raise the pH level, your duodenum secretes a peptide hormone called cholecystokinin, which causes your gallbladder to contract, releasing bile into your duodenum. That bile partially neutralizes the acidity of the chyme. Along with pancreatic enzymes, bile helps digest carbohydrates, fats, and proteins and sends these macronutrients into your small intestine for further breakdown into absorbable molecules and proper absorption of their individual nutrient components—monosaccharides from carbohydrates, amino acids from proteins, fatty acids and glycerol from fats.

Your duodenum also produces the hormone secretin, which stimulates your pancreas to release fluid that contains a high concentration of bicarbonate. This fluid, along with bile, further neutralizes gastric juices, raising chyme's pH level before it reaches the rest of your small intestine, the jejunum and ileum. When food particles are broken down just right, they're absorbed by your intestinal wall and transported to your bloodstream.

Some food material is passed from your small intestine to your large intestine, where bacteria continue to break down the proteins and starches that still aren't fully digested. When all of the nutrients are absorbed from the chyme, the remaining waste material changes into semisolids called feces and is released from your body through your rectum.

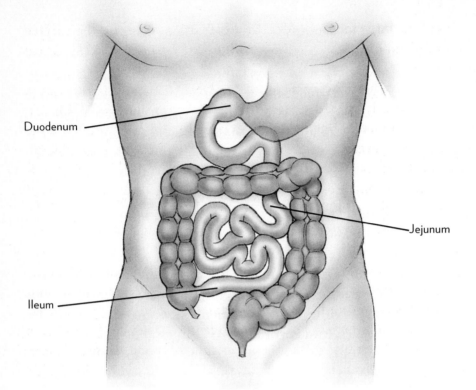

Duodenum

Jejunum

Ileum

In addition, bile removes toxins and waste products that result from the breakdown of red blood cells during a process called *catabolism*. About one-third of fecal matter is made up of dead intestinal bacteria. Your body can function smoothly and efficiently only when your bowel removes these waste products daily.

When things aren't working quite right, your body can't absorb nutrients into your blood and your cells don't get the fuel they need. The consequences? Low energy and major food cravings.

Bile plays an important role in supplying your body with fuel. It emulsifies (breaks down) fats and facilitates their digestion in your small intestine. Why do those fats have to be emulsified? It's because the enzymes that break down fat, called lipases, can't access the insides of the large fat molecules. Emulsification increases the surface area of fat, making it available for digestion by hardworking lipase enzymes.

Digestion of healthy fats is important because those fats are vital to many of your body's processes. They're necessary for the production of a group of hormonelike chemicals called prostaglandins. Prostaglandins are essential for every single cell in your body to function. They nourish and support your body's cardiovascular, reproductive, immune, and central nervous systems. Healthy fats are also essential for the absorption of calcium and the fat-soluble vitamins—A, D, E, and K.

Bile salts are essential for the absorption of both calcium and these life-essential fats in your intestines. Once bile salts have emulsified fat for absorption, they continue their journey through your small intestine, where most of them are reabsorbed into your blood within the ileum and transported back to your liver via the portal vein. There, they're collected again in bile and secreted into your duodenum. The net effect of this recirculation? Each bile salt molecule is reused about 20 times, often two or three times during a single digestive phase. Your body knows all about recycling.

Sometimes, however, this amazing recycling system is thrown off track when your intestines get congested. Congested intestines, which often lead to constipation, inhibit the recirculation of bile salts back to your liver, which slows down bile production—and that impairs the digestive process, especially after you've eaten unhealthy fats and fat-laden foods.

Why is the right amount of bile so important? When your liver produces less bile, your food may be less efficiently digested. Partially digested food may require greater quantities of hydrochloric acid (HCl) in your stomach. When your body can't produce enough HCl, food sits in your stomach and ferments, sending stomach acid upward into your esophagus and causing irritation and even injury to the delicate tissues lining it, as well as causing complications up and down your GI tract.

The result? Esophageal reflux (heartburn), which begins with a back-washing of waste, toxins, and bile from your intestines into your stomach.

Your Liver Is Your Body's Command Center

When it comes to regulating hormone levels in your bloodstream, you can count on your liver. Hormones are created by your endocrine system—one of the main networks that controls and coordinates your body's functions. Hormones interact with your nervous system, reproductive system, kidneys, gut, liver, and fat cells to facilitate communication between them and help maintain important systems and functions, including:

- Your body's energy levels

- Your reproductive system

- Your body's growth and development

- Your salt and water retention

- Your body's propensity toward internal balance, known as homeostasis

- Your responses to surroundings, stress, and injury

Specific glands and organs supply hormones directly into your blood for use inside your body in order for your endocrine system to accomplish these tasks. Your body also has exocrine glands, which secrete hormones into ducts that reach outside your body, such as salivary glands.

Endocrine glands and endocrine-related organs are very efficient worksites. They create, store, and secrete hormones as they're needed, transporting them through your bloodstream to specific targets, such as organs, tissues, or cells. For your entire endocrine system to function normally, your body needs to have at least four key things in place.

- Endocrine glands that perform correctly

- A blood supply that moves hormones efficiently to their target organs, tissues, or cells

- Receptors on the target cells for the hormones to do their work

- A system that manages hormone levels in your bloodstream, detoxifying used or completed hormones while your brain regulates hormones

Your body makes hormones from cholesterol, body fat, and other substances circulating through your bloodstream. Ideally, your body's supply of hormones is continually replenished, with new hormones entering your bloodstream as old and used hormones are detoxed, removed from your blood, and eliminated by your liver, kidneys, and large intestine.

It's a vitally important job. When your liver is clean and working efficiently, hormone levels in your blood can more easily stay balanced. But if your liver becomes congested and unable to break down, detoxify, and eliminate used hormones, they accumulate in your blood and can cause both swelling and water retention. Ironically, fluid retention plays an essential role in your body: Fluids help collect and neutralize toxins that your liver can no longer remove, thus helping protect overweight and obese people from a potentially lethal toxic crisis, such as a heart attack, septic poisoning, or massive infection. Fluid retention is a way your body protects itself from inflammation. But liver congestion leads to a vicious cycle: Your body retains water due to inflammation and food reactions. Toxins and harmful waste accumulate within the fluids around your body, further congesting the pathways of circulation and elimination, and the whole cycle begins again.

The Bottom Line

The health of your liver determines your overall health and well-being. Your liver supports your immune system in neutralizing toxins. It fuels your body. It manufactures proteins. It makes bile. And it regulates hormones. When your liver is strong and clear, it helps maintain homeostasis. On the flip side, when your body's capacity to store toxins and harmful waste is exceeded, your liver becomes overloaded. When that happens, your immune system becomes overburdened and your defenses break down. Then it's easy to get sick.

In the next chapter, you'll learn how to determine just how well—or poorly—your liver is functioning.

The LiverUp! Diaries

CINDY BROTEN, 60

The Art of Living Healthfully

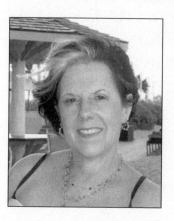

Joint pain: Reduced

Sugar cravings: Disappeared

I'm an artist with a studio in my home. I work mostly in clay, building pieces by hand—everything from mosaic tiles to vessels and sculptures. You never know exactly how a piece will turn out until it has been fired, so I've learned not to have a whole lot of expectations—sometimes things turn out completely different than you expect, and that's a good lesson in learning to live with uncertainty!

But doing this kind of work is hard on my back, and I've always had joint pain, especially in my shoulders and knees. And when I don't eat right, my symptoms seem to get worse. Last summer, I think I overindulged in sugar, wine, and processed foods—and I paid the price. I felt bloated and put on some weight, and I was having a hard time getting up in the morning and making it all the way through the day. I felt so sluggish. I learned that if I don't eat well, I don't feel well—and I really don't sleep well, either.

So I bit the bullet and followed the cleanse, and things began to improve. I think that a lot of my joint pain comes from inflammation, which I was feeding with all the sugar I'd been eating. But when I began eating well and putting healthy foods in my body, my joint pain subsided.

Since the cleanse, I've been less stiff in the morning—I can get up and get moving a lot more easily. For me, it's so doable. I end up with more energy, and I'm much more productive. The cleanse puts me on a better, healthier path.

CHAPTER 2

How Toxic Are You?

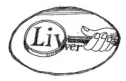

Even if you've been feeling under the weather, chances are your doctor's never mentioned anything about the health of your liver. But as you'll learn in this chapter, when your liver's not up to speed, the rest of your body isn't, either.

One of the reasons we pay so little attention to the liver is that conventional blood tests that doctors use routinely to check it aren't very sensitive. These tests check for liver damage, rather than liver function. Liver damage is determined by a rise in liver enzymes, known as aminotransferase enzymes, including aspartate aminotransferase (AST or SGOT) and alanine aminotransferase (ALT or SGPT). Normally, these enzymes are predominantly contained within liver cells and, to a lesser degree, muscle cells. But if your liver is injured or damaged, it leaks these enzymes into your blood, raising the levels of AST and ALT in your blood—and signaling liver disease.

The problem is, these raised liver enzymes are found in your blood only *after* they've been released because of damage. So even if your blood tests for liver enzymes and liver proteins are normal, your liver may not be working at its best for you to feel really well.

If, after reading this chapter, you suspect that your liver isn't working optimally, you may want to ask your physician to check it. CT scans, MRI scans, and ultrasounds can reveal the size, texture, and shape of your liver, along with other organs in your upper abdomen. Blood tests can check bilirubin levels that can help determine liver health. If your liver enzymes are high, damage has already occurred, but all is not lost.

The liver is an amazing, resilient organ that can be rehabilitated and detoxified.

At some point, you've probably experienced some vague symptoms for which your doctor can't seem to find a cause. Maybe you've felt under par after overdoing it—after the holidays or celebrations when you've consumed too much sugar, caffeine, alcohol, or processed food or just too much food in general. Or you may have sensed that something was off after being exposed to toxins like mold or being in a place that had been treated chemically—from public washrooms to lawns to entire neighborhoods during mosquito season. Whatever the cause, you've probably experienced times when your body had to work hard to detoxify itself.

How Toxic Is Your Liver?

When the toxin level in your body exceeds your liver's capacity to detoxify, you can experience a range of symptoms that point to a sluggish or toxic liver. The following quiz will help you think about whether or not your liver could use a cleaning. Answer the questions before and after you complete the LiverUp! Cleanse in Chapter 5. It's a simple 12-day program designed to detox, heal, and rejuvenate your body's hardest-working organ, boosting your liver's ability to detox itself both by reducing your intake of toxins and by supplying it with foods that boost its detox potential.

{The Healthy Liver Quiz

Do you suffer regular headaches or migraines? _____

Do you suffer from sinus issues, such as excessive
mucus, stuffy nose, or hay fever? _____

Do you have dark circles under your eyes? _____

Do you have red, swollen, or itchy eyes? _____

Do you have skin issues, such as acne, itchy rashes,
hives, or general dermatitis? _____

Do you experience joint pain; arthritis; puffy feet, ankles, or hands; or inflamation? _____

Do you have excessive body heat or heavy perspiration? _____

Do you have strong body odor? _____

Do you wake up with a coated tongue, a bitter taste in your mouth, or bad breath? _____

Do you suffer from bloating, gas, indigestion, or nausea, particularly after eating fatty foods? _____

Do you suffer from constipation or diarrhea? _____

Do you experience sugar cravings, mood swings, fuzzy thinking, difficulty concentrating, poor memory, or depression? _____

Do you feel lethargic? _____

Do you have difficulty controlling your weight, even when you eat less? _____

Do you suffer from high blood pressure or high cholesterol? _____

Do you experience hormonal imbalances, such as PMS or hot flashes? _____

Do you have a strong reaction to the effects of alcohol or coffee? _____

TOTAL SCORE _____

YOUR LIVER HEALTH SCORECARD

8 OR MORE YES RESPONSES: Your liver is having an impact on your overall health and well-being, and a liver detox is in order.

5-7 YES RESPONSES: You're beginning to experience symptoms of an overburdened liver. You need to reduce your liver load; liver detox will help.

0-4 YES RESPONSES: It's unlikely you have issues with your liver's detox process, but everyone can benefit from a liver detox.

If you have any of these symptoms, you may be suffering from a sluggish or toxic liver. Don't be discouraged by the number of symptoms you're experiencing. After all, day in and day out, your body is besieged by toxins, and your liver is the clearinghouse for most all of them. When it can't keep pace with the rate and level of these inflowing toxins, your body stores them in your fat cells. And as we've already learned, your body retains fluid and creates fat cells to accommodate these unprocessed toxins as a way to protect your organs and tissues.

But when toxins remain, your body literally becomes "intoxicated" and begins to manifest a wide array of problems. Yet while your liver must work overtime to filter all the toxins that bombard your body, it can rehabilitate itself if you take a few steps toward cleaning and healing it. That's what this book is all about—leading you through the steps necessary for healing and restoring your liver and living a healthier, happier life.

Your Medical Conditions and Your Liver

Let's look at the role your liver plays in many health conditions. Here's a quick look at some of the health problems that may come about when your liver isn't working at its best.

Headaches

Almost everyone has an occasional headache. If it's infrequent and mild, you probably just take some aspirin or ibuprofen and carry on. But if you suffer from persistent headaches, it's a good idea to explore what might be triggering them.

Headaches can be either muscular or vascular in nature, and both types are affected by your liver. Muscular headaches are caused by increased tension, particularly in and around your head. This tension can be caused by any number of factors, from eye strain (caused by squinting in the sun or hours spent reading) and neck strain (caused by hours spent in front of the computer) to emotional stress, fatigue, or high blood pressure. At times, you may suffer several conditions simultaneously, thus almost ensuring a headache.

Accrued toxins and compromised digestion due to toxins can also cause muscle tension. Some foods seem to be particularly problematic and likely to trigger muscular headaches, such as red wine, cheese, and chocolate. Other triggers include certain scents found in perfumes and laundry detergents, along with fumes from solvents and various cleaning products. Ongoing muscle tension creates pain.

You can also experience vascular headaches, which result when the blood vessels of your head either constrict or dilate too much. Toxins such as solvents (nail polish remover and paint thinner), hormonal fluctuations, and caffeine can trigger these headaches.

Caffeine plays a dual role in headaches. It can trigger or tame them— or both. Overindulgence can lead to tightening of your blood vessels, as muscles in the walls of your blood vessels constrict and accumulate lactic acid—and that creates pain. Or a headache can happen after drinking lots of coffee, as your body craves more caffeine. Or, the blood vessels in your head may dilate, extending the miniscule nerves that flank your blood vessels and causing pain—and sometimes you may grab a cup of coffee just to counteract that feeling.

Migraines

Migraines tend to occur when blood vessels in your head become dilated for an extended period of time, often because of these factors: genes, stress, and a trigger—a food sensitivity, too much estrogen, or an allergy. When this happens, your liver isn't able to efficiently process, transform, and eliminate toxins. The result: Toxins build up in your blood, dilating your blood vessels, which leads to pain and throbbing.

Estrogen dominance—the theory that some health problems occur when there's too much estrogen and not enough progesterone in your body—seems to play a role in migraines. And one of the big factors leading to estrogen dominance? Stress. In stressful situations, your body produces the stress hormone cortisol, which raises your estrogen levels. That starts a cascade of problems. Too much estrogen leads to fluid retention and weight gain. And that extra estrogen goes looking for fat cells for storage. So the more estrogen you retain, the more weight you may gain—and both the estrogen and the weight compromise your liver. After all, your body produces estrogen regularly for many important functions. So when your liver is overloaded with toxins, it can't filter and eliminate estrogen properly, leading to many health problems, including migraine headaches.[1]

Plus, external estrogens—xenoestrogens—further compromise your liver and can trigger migraines. Xenoestrogens are everywhere—from pesticides to plastics, from car exhaust to household cleaners, from cosmetics and beauty products to carpeting and furniture. These chemicals create mayhem with your hormones, overload your liver, and cause a myriad of health challenges, including migraines.[2]

Sinus Issues, Allergies, and Skin Complaints

Your liver harbors immune cells that filter toxins and synthetic chemicals found in your food (artificial flavorings, sweeteners, colorings, and preservatives) from your blood as it travels through your liver for cleaning. When your liver is compromised, though, foreign particles and chemicals like these flow back into your bloodstream and find their way into the cells of various organs, muscles, and joints. Your body considers these foreign particles to be pathogens and kicks into action, creating antibodies that attack its own cells. That's how your body's immune system can be fooled into attacking the very cells it's meant to support and protect. With your immune system hyperalert, your body produces mucus and inflammation unremittingly. This ongoing immune response can initiate allergies and flulike symptoms.

Like your liver, your skin is also a detox organ. When your liver is overburdened and weakened, your skin will pick up the slack and try to eliminate toxins, causing a variety of symptoms such as skin rashes, acne, dermatitis, and liver spots. Since your liver is your body's major blood filter, when it's not functioning optimally, those toxins that remain in your body create free radicals, which promote cell damage in your skin.[3]

Tissue Swelling, Joint Pain, Stiffness, Arthritis, Inflammation, and Body Heat

Back in Chapter 1, we learned that both blood proteins and hormones regulate healthy fluid balances in your body. Your liver makes two of these essential blood proteins—albumins and globulins, both of which are critical in maintaining proper fluid balance between your blood and your tissue. Blood proteins in your capillary beds—one-cell-thick vessels—can't flow from the capillary beds into the surrounding tissue because they're too big. So blood fluid is pulled into the capillary beds from the tissue.

Swelling. But if your liver is overloaded and can't produce enough blood proteins—or can't process them efficiently—the result is edema, or tissue swelling, which happens when there's not enough pressure to pull fluid back from these tissues and into your blood. This fluid is mainly seen in the ankles and legs, yet fluid retention can occur throughout your body and can cause a variety of symptoms, including fatigue. If left untreated, edema can lead to difficulty walking, decreased blood circulation, skin ulcers, and infections.

Joint Pain, Stiffness, Arthritis, and Inflammation. Most joint pain involves inflammation—either local, affecting one specific part of your body, or systemic, affecting your entire body. When you experience an injury, your immune system triggers a series of events known as the inflammatory cascade—inflammatory hormones are released to activate your white blood cells, which then restore damaged tissue and clear out infection. This inflammation causes the redness, swelling, and pain that follows an injury.

Once the immediate threat is addressed and your body seeks equilibrium, anti-inflammatory compounds take over to heal the injured area. It's a sign of a healthy immune system when local or acute inflammation diminishes. But when the symptoms of inflammation don't disappear, your body's immune system may have gone into overdrive, causing more general inflammation.

We've already learned that the toxic chemicals your liver can't transform or neutralize eventually leak into your bloodstream and tissues. And when those toxic compounds build up, your immune system attacks them as pathogens, triggering inflammation. In this hyperactive state, inflammation accumulates in the surrounding tissues of your joints, creating swelling, stiffness, and pain.

Research shows that chronic stress weakens your immune system, inhibiting its ability to regulate itself. Ongoing stress prompts the continual release of cortisol, which not only creates inflammation, but also fuels existing inflammation. In this proinflammatory environment, hormone communication with your brain breaks down, so your brain doesn't get the message that the trouble is over and no more cortisol is needed. The result is that your stressed-out body and mind live in a continual state of emergency—or chronic inflammation—and that can even lead to pain and swelling in your joints. A study at Washington University in St. Louis measured the level of inflammation in parents whose children were undergoing treatment for pediatric cancer. Researchers examined what happens to people's immune systems during ongoing stressful situations by comparing 25 healthy parents whose children were undergoing treatment for pediatric cancer with 25 healthy parents of healthy children, focusing on measures of mental health and immune system responses. All of the parents had blood drawn at the initial session and cortisol samples taken over 2 days. The findings: Parents of cancer patients reported more psychological distress than parents of healthy children. The parents of cancer patients also showed less response to glucocorticoid, the hormone that slows down the production of the proinflammatory chemicals.

The study confirmed that chronic stress appears to weaken the immune system's ability to respond to those hormones, which help shut down the body's inflammatory response after infection or injury. Researchers think psychological stress may start—or continue—inflammatory conditions like allergies and autoimmune, cardiovascular, infectious, and rheumatologic diseases.[4]

Excessive Body Heat, Perspiration, and Odor. Excess body heat, often with perspiration and body odor, can signal a toxic liver. When your liver is overworked, it expands. Struggling toward equilibrium, it generates heat, often causing your whole body to overheat.

Traditional Chinese medicine holds that excess heat in people who consume a rich diet (including excess fats, proteins, and sugary products) is often related to liver excess. Your liver heats up and expands as it attempts to process, transform, or eliminate toxic chemicals from your environment and your food. Seeking equilibrium, your body sweats as it tries to eliminate toxins by excreting them through your skin and to cool down its inner temperature. Offensive body odor often directly correlates to the toxins your body is trying to eliminate.[5]

Digestive Issues

Coated Tongue and Bad Breath. Eastern medicine has known for thousands of years that your tongue reflects digestive and liver health. Often a coated tongue indicates mucus, which points to poor digestion, or a liver overburdened by toxins. When your digestion is compromised, bacteria from your bowel and yeast (such as *Candida*) may be present. The culprits may be mucus-causing foods such as dairy, excessive fats, sugar, alcohol, and processed foods, which burden your liver and result in pro-inflammatory health issues. Bad breath can also result from a compromised digestion system and overloaded liver.[6]

Bloating, Gas, Indigestion, Constipation, or Diarrhea. Your liver is also a digestive organ, serving two essential purposes: filtration and bile production. It filters out those chemicals (exotoxins and endotoxins) that are dangerous to your body while transforming or eliminating nutrients you've consumed in excess.

As your liver aids in the digestion, assimilation, and excretion of your food, it secretes filtered toxins into one of two substances—urea or bile. When your liver breaks down proteins, it creates the leftover waste into ammonia, which the liver breaks down further to urea so the body can remove it. In an effort to excrete by-product waste and toxins, your liver transport urea from your blood to your kidneys. In addition to removing wastes, bile, which is stored in your gallbladder, also helps break down fats so your body can absorb and assimilate them. Then it transports waste by-products and toxins filtered from your liver into your intestines for elimination.

Your liver is a key player in the digestive process, taking on double duty. When you consume fatty foods, bile is released from your gallbladder into your intestines to break down those fats. The nutrients from these foods travel to the capillaries in your intestines and are absorbed into your blood stream. This nutrient-rich blood flows into the portal vein, which transports digested food from your small intestine back to your liver. Your liver helps to both metabolize nutrients and filter toxins, then sends nutrient-rich blood back into your body to feed your cells. It is here that those toxins and excess by-products are converted into urea and bile. Urea travels to your kidneys, and it's then excreted via urine. Once it's dumped wastes into the intestine for elimination, bile from your liver is stored in your gallbladder until it's needed to break down fats and eliminate wastes in your intestines as the digestive process is continually working—often overtime.

When that happens—if your liver is overworked and can't produce enough bile—your body can't emulsify fats efficiently and doesn't make them water soluble to allow your body to absorb and assimilate them. Without proper amounts of bile, your body dumps fats into your large intestine for elimination, lessening the process of absorption. With less absorption, your body can't get those essential fats that enable it to absorb vitamins A, D, E, and K. These fat-soluble vitamins support your immune system, preserve muscle tone, boost energy, and maintain healthy skin, hair, gums, and vision.

Bile also lubricates and stimulates your digestive tract, so insufficient amounts can result in constipation, indigestion, gas, bloating, and irritable bowel syndrome, triggering both constipation and diarrhea. And when your bowels finally do move, the stools can be light colored, containing greasy, undigested fat.[7]

Blood Sugar Issues

Since your liver must filter, transform, or neutralize most everything you consume, it can really get overworked when your diet is largely made up of processed carbohydrates like cereal, bread, pasta, and baked goods. Unlike fresh, whole foods (vegetables, fruits, nuts, seeds, and whole grains), processed foods and drinks are often stripped of nutrients and loaded with added chemicals, additives, sugar, high-fructose corn syrup, and preservatives—and filtering all of that is a burden on your liver.

Unfortunately, processed carbohydrates and sugar-laden foods and drinks make up the standard American diet (SAD). For many North Americans, a day's menu might look something like this:

- A large coffee and an oversized muffin for breakfast

- Pizza and soda for lunch

- Pasta with cream sauce and a glass of wine for dinner

- Some snacks in between, such as crackers or a cookie

Sound familiar? Where are the fresh, vital foods that don't contain added chemicals? Those are the foods your body needs, and they keep your liver happier. For both your liver and your pancreas, the standard high-carb diet is a nightmare. These organs have to work overtime to process those chemical-infused, refined foods, and at some point, both

organs weaken under the stress—and your body experiences the consequences in a variety of ways.

When your diet consists of wholesome, nourishing foods, enabling
your liver and pancreas to maintain steady blood sugar levels throughout
your day, you experience health and vitality. Here's what that looks like:

- Your thinking is clear.
- You're awake and aware.

{Sugar Central

Just a quick look at the part your liver plays in digestion will show you why it's so
important to look after this vital organ. During digestion, your body breaks
down all of the carbs you've consumed into their simplest form—glucose—and
releases this fuel into your bloodstream. When this happens, your pancreas
senses a sharp increase in blood sugar and sends a signal for insulin to move to
the surface of cells throughout your body. Insulin helps pull glucose from your
blood and into your cells, where it can be used for energy.

Insulin is a gatekeeper for glucose at the cellular level. Every cell in your
body, from your brain to your baby toe, uses glucose as energy to function. And
for your cells to use this energy, they need insulin, which allows the glucose to
pass through your cell walls.[8]

If your cells can't use all the glucose in your blood, your liver converts the
excess glucose into glycogen and stores it right there in your liver until it's
needed. But your liver can only store so much. When it has reached its tipping
point, your liver begins to convert all the glucose it has absorbed from your
blood into fatty acids, known as triglycerides, and cholesterol, which your body,
in turn, stores as fat. Some of this fat gets stored in fat tissues (increasing your
fat and weight), and some of the cholesterol may even get deposited on the
insides of the walls of your blood vesssels.[9]

When your blood sugar levels drop or you need energy and you don't have
food/fuel being processed, your liver converts this stored glycogen back into
glucose and releases it into your bloodstream for your cells to use as energy.
This give-and-take process within your liver helps your body maintain
homeostasis—that's the process by which your body works to maintain a state of
physiological balance so it can stay alive and healthy.

- You can focus and concentrate at work and play.

- Your mood is even, with no major peaks right after eating and no valleys hours later.

- You don't crave sugar, caffeine, or processed snack foods to sustain your energy.

But when your diet consists of foods that are stripped of nutrients and full of sugars like high-fructose corn syrup (HFCS), your pancreas goes into overdrive, pumping lots of insulin into your blood. And when that happens, the results are predictable.

- Your blood sugar levels and energy come crashing down, often leading to agitation.

- Excess glucose gets stored as glycogen in your liver.

- Excess glycogen is turned into fat within your liver, which can trigger insulin resistance.

That adds up to a condition called nonalcoholic fatty liver disease (NAFLD), which means your normal, healthy liver tissue is replaced, in part, with areas of unhealthy fats.

What's so bad about that? A couple of things. When your liver becomes fatty, it can't respond properly to insulin. Even though there's plenty of insulin circulating around your body, your overburdened liver can't respond until insulin levels rise even higher. The result is insulin resistance. And when your cells become insulin resistant, it takes much more insulin than usual to push that circulating glucose into them.

And that's not all. When your cells become insulin resistant, a vicious cycle gets set in motion, which can lead to a couple of other serious conditions.

First, your pancreas responds to rising blood sugar by pumping out more and more insulin. Eventually your pancreas can no longer keep up with the demand and, worn out with the effort, succumbs to "pancreatic exhaustion." Second, your liver becomes puzzled by the lackluster insulin response to rising glucose levels in your bloodstream. Assuming the glucose is a sign that your blood sugar is too low, your liver dumps even *more* glucose into your bloodstream.

Sounds complicated? It is. All of this metabolic confusion can cause sugar cravings, fuzzy thinking, difficulty concentrating, poor memory, and mood swings. High blood sugar—that's when your cells can't extract glucose from your blood—can make you feel drowsy, lethargic, weak, and even exhausted. High blood sugar levels can leave you hungry, unable to concentrate, confused, emotionally volatile—and absolutely *craving* sugar.

Then there's low blood sugar. That's when a big drop in blood sugar levels leaves you craving more sugar. Low blood sugar levels affect your ability to concentrate, to focus, and to think clearly. Low blood sugar levels can leave you feeling restless, irritable, and depressed.

So what does all of this add up to? It's simple: When your liver can't process significant quantities of refined carbohydrates, you experience similar symptoms with both high and low blood sugar.

Toxicity Issues and Your Brain

When your liver is sluggish, even your brain is affected. Excessive amounts of toxic substances, finding their way into your bloodstream, can affect the way your brain functions. Toxic blood flowing into your brain can generate "foggy brain," impaired concentration and memory, unpleasant mood swings, and even depression.

Some of this toxicity is generated in your gut when by-products are formed from yeast overgrowth. In advanced cases of liver disease, ammonia by-products affect brain chemistry.

Besides distributing energy to each and every one of your cells, one of your liver's primary jobs is to clean your blood. But when it's weak and working inefficiently, it can't detoxify your blood effectively. That's problematic because when your blood is encumbered with toxins, it can't easily carry oxygen and nutrients to your cells. Since every cell in your body needs oxygen and nutrients to function, those low levels can leave you feeling chronically fatigued and lethargic.

When things are working as they should, your liver produces cleaner blood, which carries more oxygen and nutrients. Clean blood is also lighter—it flows better, circulating to all of your extremities more efficiently, energizing every cell in your body—all the more reason to support a clean and efficient liver.

Weight-Control Issues

Since your liver is your body's primary fat-burning organ, a clean, healthy liver is key to reaching and maintaining a healthy weight. With a diet loaded with processed carbs and unhealthy fats, an environment filled with pollutants, and synthetic chemicals hidden in your foods and your homes, it's no surprise that your liver might not be as healthy as it should be and weight is so tough to control—despite your best efforts. When toxins accrue in your body, they stress your liver, clog your colon, and accumulate as fat.

When you overload your body with toxins and pollutants, you create a toxic liver—and a toxic liver will sabotage any weight-loss efforts. In these conditions, your liver, working overtime to detoxify your body, cannot metabolize fat. The result? Your liver dumps fat and cholesterol back into your bloodstream, disrupting weight loss and potentially causing even more health problems.

High Blood Pressure and High Cholesterol

The liver and its functions are tied in with factors that contribute to various cardiovascular problems. High blood pressure and high cholesterol play a critical role in determining these medical conditions.

High Blood Pressure. Remember what happens when your liver gets flooded with glucose: It goes into conservation mode and tries to store as much glycogen as possible. Excess glycogen in your liver gets converted into fatty acids in your liver's tissues. And when these tissues become infiltrated with fat, normal liver enzymes change or become elevated. By the time your liver enzymes are altered or elevated, your distressed liver has begun to affect your blood and heart.

Research has shown that disrupted liver enzymes are linked to the development of high blood pressure. A study at the State University of New York at Buffalo confirmed that accumulation of fat in the liver is linked with hypertension. The study involved 1,455 participants who were tested for liver enzymes, blood pressure, weight, and size of waistline.

At the 6-year follow-up, participants were divided into five groups according to their baseline enzyme levels. Participants had their baseline levels measured again and then were asked to complete questionnaires about their lifestyles and behaviors, including their use of alcohol. Participants with increased central body fat and nonalcoholic fatty liver showed higher levels of hypertension. These findings suggest that fatty liver is linked to metabolic syndrome, a set of symptoms that point to the risk for cardiovascular disease.[10]

That's not all. A fatty liver puts stress on another major filtering organ: your kidneys. Scientists have determined that a diseased liver impacts kidney function, leading to a cascade of negative consequences. A study in the *Journal of the American Society of Nephrology* reports that in patients with type 2 diabetes, nonalcoholic fatty liver disease (NAFLD) or "fatty liver" may pose an important risk factor for diabetes-related chronic kidney disease (CKD).

In the study, conducted at the University of Verona, the relationship between NAFLD and CKD was examined in 1,760 adult patients with type 2 diabetes, all of whom initially had normal or near-normal kidney function. Over the next 6½ years, 547 patients developed CKD, with a yearly risk of about 4.5 percent. According to lead scientists, the risk of CKD was 69 percent higher for patients with fatty liver than for those without it. This study suggests that a fatty liver may release pathogens—pro-inflammatory chemicals—that contribute to diabetic kidney damage.[11]

Since your kidneys control your blood pressure, whatever affects your kidneys affects your blood pressure too. If your liver affects your kidneys, damage to your liver can cause damage to your kidneys, raising your blood pressure. This connection might explain why obesity, diabetes, high cholesterol, and high blood sugar—along with alcohol abuse—are risk factors for high blood pressure. In turn, each of these factors is also a risk factor for fatty liver.[12] It's all connected.

Finally, a toxic liver can't break down the adrenal hormone aldosterone, which increases blood volume in your body and raises blood pressure. It also balances electrolytes in your blood, distributes fluids, and retains needed salt throughout your body. That balance of fluids and salt retention helps control blood pressure. Aldosterone also helps remove excess potassium, keeping those levels balanced. When your liver is overburdened and can't break down aldosterone, the hormone accumulates in your body, making you retain excess sodium and lowering your potassium levels—the combined effects of which raise blood pressure.

High Cholesterol. Besides regulating fat metabolism by burning or eliminating fat, your liver manufactures and distributes cholesterol throughout your body. Cholesterol is a waxy fat substance that is an essential component of every cell in your body, helping to maintain cellular structure and membranes. In addition, cholesterol helps cells communicate with one another, enabling whole systems to work together. While each cell makes cholesterol, cells often need more than they can make themselves. Your liver then produces and transports extra cholesterol to your cells.

These fat-soluble substances need a transport vehicle—known as LDL ("bad") cholesterol—to move through viscous or thick body fluids.

LDL cholesterol is large enough to transport cholesterol's smaller, fatty substances, along with dietary fat, essential fatty acids, and fat-soluble antioxidants (vitamin A, carotenes, vitamin K, coenzyme Q_{10}, and vitamin E). LDL's ability to transport cholesterol is vital to the health and survival of every cell in your body.

But there's a downside: Your liver can produce too much LDL cholesterol, primarily as a result of the standard American diet, which is filled with processed foods, excess sugar, oxidized fat, and insufficient fiber. Remember how your liver converts excess processed food into fat and then stores it? When your liver becomes saturated with fat, it creates extra LDL, packing it with fatty acids, known as triglycerides, and releasing LDL into your bloodstream to relieve itself of excess fat.

In a liver burdened by fat accumulation, the liver's cells and the spaces in between are filled with fat, making the liver slightly enlarged and heavier and giving it a yellow, greasy appearance. And this liver congestion affects the bile flow and gallbladder and makes it possible to harbor gallstones made of cholesterol and bile.

A robust liver, on the other hand, is dark pink-red, a result of healthy bloodflow in the spaces between the cells. Banks of liver cells stack to create the walls of these spaces. As blood, carrying toxins, waste by-products, and fat, flows through these spaces, the liver, acting like a giant sieve, filters and cleans your entire bloodstream. However, when the spaces and cells in your liver get congested with fat and toxins, your liver can't detox your blood efficiently or effectively.

Your liver is the major fat-burning organ in your body. It not only burns fat but also helps to pump excessive fat out of your body, by way of bile that moves into your intestines for elimination. If your liver is healthy, managing both weight and fat accumulation is easy. But a fatty liver stores extra fat instead of burning and removing it, thus turning itself into a warehouse for stored fat and a distribution center for excess cholesterol that will be deposited all over your body. Some of this cholesterol ends up stuck inside the walls of your arteries, leading to serious consequences for your health and well-being.[13]

Hormonal Imbalances and Menstrual Issues, Menopausal Disturbances, and Hot Flashes

You already know that your liver is a busy—and very important—organ. Among its many responsibilities: regulating hormone levels in your bloodstream. Your body makes hormones continually, to control virtually all of its functions: growth, reproduction, metabolism, and weight.

Your hormones, produced in your endocrine glands, carry information and instructions to various parts of your body, enabling them to communicate with one another. These hormones have subtle and powerful actions and yet are sensitive to many chemicals. Given the amount of toxins in the environment and in your food, your hormonal system is particularly vulnerable. That's because:

- We consume foods loaded with hormones, created to speed the growth process for animals in preparation for slaughter. In turn, we eat the meat and drink the milk from these animals. Milk, the basis of all dairy products, is particularly high in added hormones.

- Within your own body, those tissues that produce hormones contain a large percentage of fat and have a rich supply of blood, so they easily accumulate fat-soluble toxins traveling through your bloodstream.

- Xenoestrogens (false estrogens; see page 40 for more information) mimic the behavior of natural hormones, but unlike natural hormones that can respond to signals from your brain, these false hormones can't regulate themselves.

- Toxins and chemicals can inhibit cell receptors of natural hormones by embedding between the hormones and the tissues they need to stimulate, thus preventing natural hormones from doing their jobs. Moreover, these toxins and chemicals can impair the natural rhythm of hormonal release, interrupting millions of subsequent natural reactions in your body.

In addition to affecting hormones directly, toxins also affect your liver's ability to regulate these hormones. As your body continually replenishes its supply of hormones, your liver, along with your kidneys, removes used hormones from your blood. When your liver is working efficiently, regulating hormone levels in your blood is a snap. But when it's overloaded and unable to eliminate used hormones, they accumulate in your blood, disrupting your body's ability to function effectively. Xenoestrogens in particular—found in weight-promoting animal feed, household chemicals, birth control pills, hormone replacement therapy (HRT), and cosmetics—interfere with natural hormones in your body and contribute to the dominance of estrogen (the female hormone that's connected to menstruation, pregnancy, and menopause) that stimulates cell growth in both women and men.

Estrogen dominance, from both natural and chemical-based estrogen, has been linked to many unpleasant symptoms related to menstruation and perimenopause, including breast tenderness, PMS, headaches, irregular periods, and hot flashes. Estrogen may also play a role in female cancers, which result from unrestrained cell growth in a woman's breasts, uterus, or ovaries.[14]

Sensitivity to Alcohol and Caffeine

Alcohol and caffeine require your liver to work especially hard. But when your liver is congested, it can't metabolize alcohol or caffeine efficiently. As a result, your body becomes sensitive to their effects.

Alcohol. Alcohol, one of the most distilled forms of sugar, is so absorbable that you feel its effects in your brain within minutes. It acts like sugar on steroids, raising blood sugar levels initially, then acting like a depressant. It takes a big toll on your liver. Here's how: Your body readily absorbs alcohol from your gastrointestinal tract, but since alcohol can't be stored, it has to be oxidized and eliminated. And your liver is the only organ that can do the job, by mobilizing its enzymes and performing several metabolic conversions.

First, it must convert the ethanol in alcohol to acetaldehyde, using an enzyme called acetaldehyde oxidase. Then, acetaldehyde molecules are metabolized into acetic acid radicals. Finally, these acetic acid radicals are broken down into carbon dioxide and water so your body can excrete them.

If your liver is congested and its enzymes are underfunctioning, it can't finish the oxidation process. The result is that excess acetaldehyde, a highly acidic poison that's closely related to formaldehyde,[15] circulates throughout your body. When it accumulates, your blood becomes acidic with toxins and you end up with acidosis, also known as a hangover, complete with nausea, headache, brain fog, or stomach upset. Nearly 80 years ago, a physician named Dr. William Hay, considered by many to be the "father" of pH theory, asserted that acidosis may be the leading cause of premature aging and can lead to weight gain, fatty liver, and heart attack.[16] His research and insight are even more relevant today.

In addition to leaving you with uncomfortable hangovers, an overloaded liver can also lower your body's tolerance to alcohol. In a condition called reverse tolerance, your liver can no longer produce enough enzymes to break down alcohol effectively. When your body can no longer metabolize alcohol well, you can get very intoxicated on small quantities—much less than is needed to affect a person who rarely drinks.

A small percentage of the general population is diagnosed with a genetic enzyme disorder called Gilbert's syndrome (GS), which affects enzymes that help metabolize bilirubin (a breakdown product of hemoglobin), alcohol, and Tylenol. GS affects the body's ability to detoxify and conjugate both endogenous and exogenous toxins, and that results in pigment recirculating through the body, creating a slight yellowing tinge to the skin, known as jaundice. Scientists are learning that this "benign" condition is actually a deeper issue that requires some lifestyle adaptations. Some people with GS report symptoms of chronic fatigue and headaches, symptoms that appear to point toward a toxic liver. People with GS should limit their alcohol and acetaminophen (Tylenol) use.

Alcohol also interferes with estrogen metabolism, causing an almost immediate hormonal imbalance and filling your blood with excess estrogen relative to progesterone. Ask any menopausal woman about the effect of drinking alcohol, and she'll likely tell you about the unwelcome onset of hot flashes. Another reason for a healthy diet: The more alcohol you consume, the more antioxidants you need to detox and strengthen your body. Vitamin C, found in all citrus, is particularly important.[17]

Caffeine. You may think of caffeine as the elixir that kick-starts your morning, but your body, which can't be fooled, greets caffeine like a toxin. While caffeine boosts mood and energy levels in the short term, your body can't sustain these levels. Within a couple of hours, your mood and energy come sliding (or crashing) down.

In *Change Your Brain, Change Your Body*, Daniel Amen, MD, suggests that caffeine disrupts your natural sleep process, involving the brain chemical adenosine and its receptors.[18] Adenosine calms your body and facilitates sleep. When it's produced in your brain, it attaches to its own adenosine receptors, causing your brain's blood vessels to dilate, most likely ensuring good oxygenation during sleep.

But caffeine interferes with this progression because it binds to these same receptors, making fewer of them available for adenosine. Instead of calming brain activity, caffeine does just the opposite, constricting your brain's blood vessels, speeding up neuronal activity, and signaling your body to go on high alert by producing adrenaline, the fight-or-flight hormone that signals your heart to pump harder, increasing blood pressure, opening airways in your lungs, and narrowing blood vessels in your skin and intestines to increase bloodflow to major muscle groups. This adrenaline surge gives you that java jolt, making your heart beat faster, your breathing become shallower, and your muscles tense up. It also boosts dopamine levels, activating your brain's pleasure centers.

Adrenaline enables your body to fight or run when encountering a perceived threat. Both adrenaline and dopamine make you feel more alert, motivated, energized, and stimulated. No wonder we love our coffee, tea, and other caffeinated drinks. But the bad news is that when the effects of the caffeine wear off, you feel sluggish, fatigued, and even depressed—so you look to more caffeine to reenergize. Soon you're hooked on the stuff, and it may take more and more to achieve that same feeling.

Caffeine's effects are felt most acutely 30 to 60 minutes after you've consumed it. That's when the chemical reaches its peak concentration and when your liver works to metabolize it. Your liver must work very hard to detoxify caffeine, directing all of its efforts toward breaking it down and leaving other toxins circulating in its tissues.

Studies have shown that serious coffee drinkers have higher levels of anxiety and depression, plus stress-related medical complications. In the United Kingdom's Optimum Nutrition survey, 55,000 people were questioned about the effects of caffeine on their physical and emotional well-being. The response: The more caffeinated drinks people consumed, the more fatigued they were. Participants reported experiencing the following symptoms with increased caffeine consumption: increased lethargy, reduced libido, fluid retention, joint stiffness, and pain. Menopausal women reported increased symptoms, like hot flashes and night sweats.[19] In *The Detox Diet* by Elson Haas, MD, excess nervousness, irritability, insomnia, restless leg syndrome, dizziness, general anxiety (and even panic attacks), and subsequent fatigue top the list of negative side effects of caffeine. Many of these signs and symptoms are associated with anxiety and depression.[20]

Caffeine also functions as a diuretic, encouraging your body to rid itself of fluids. And without sufficient fluids, toxins are reabsorbed back into your bloodstream.

Next Steps

Any of the symptoms discussed in this chapter sound familiar? If they do, you'll benefit from a liver cleanse. In fact, *everyone* can benefit from a liver cleanse. In my practice, I've supervised hundreds of people embarking on one of my seasonal cleanses. And almost every person reports a remarkable improvement. Some of the positive changes they've experienced include:

- Increased energy
- Clearer thinking
- Alertness upon waking
- Better sleep
- Better digestion
- Less water retention
- Weight loss
- Decreased hormonal symptoms
- Fewer mood swings
- Lower blood pressure

When your body is processing and releasing toxins efficiently, you feel energized, alert, and balanced. You can support your body's efforts in maintaining balance and homeostasis by detoxing in two ways: by reducing the toxins you expose your body to and by improving your body's ability to detoxify itself.

The LiverUp! 12-day cleanse offers both a reduction in the toxins you'll consume and a way to boost your body's detox potential. The result: You'll feel better within days. In the next chapter, we'll take a closer look at how your liver works and why the foods you eat play such a significant role in its health.

The LiverUp! Diaries

ELAINE BURNS, 57

I Opened Up to New Possibilities

Sinus pain: Conquered

Confidence: Increased

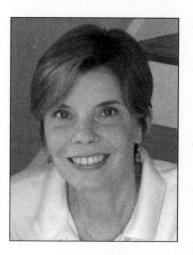

For years, I was plagued with sinus problems. I'd experience nagging headaches and terrible pressure, and my doctor would just tell me to use antihistamines or nasal sprays, or even Sudafed. But nothing seemed to work very well, and the pain kept me from doing a lot of things I would have enjoyed.

I first tried the LiverUp! Cleanse in 2010, and I followed the program exactly. I loved learning all the specifics about the foods in the cleanse and how supporting my liver could actually help me with my sinus issues. I was really careful about choosing good, healthy foods—all those crucifers; green, leafy vegetables; and citrus fruits—and staying away from stuff that stresses my liver. I think dairy and sugar were big culprits for me. The cleanse seemed to make a difference really quickly. I think my sluggish liver had been having an impact on my sinuses, but soon after I began the cleanse they really opened up. I was surprised to see how great I felt after being more intentional about the way I ate and the way I lived. I began waking up in the morning feeling excited about starting my day.

Not only did my sinuses open up, but my life opened up, too. When I started feeling better, I had so much more energy. I began exercising again after a long break, going to yoga and swimming regularly. I involved myself again in organizations that are near and dear to my heart by taking on some leadership positions that I had previously declined because I didn't feel like I had enough energy.

My sinus problems? Pretty much gone. I've modified my diet significantly from what I used to eat—now I hardly ever have sugar or processed foods. And even when I try foods that aren't so great, I'm generally eating so well that I don't get into trouble with my sinuses anymore. I've really turned it around.

CHAPTER 3

Your Liver's Two-Phase Detoxification Process

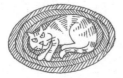

I n Chapter 1, we learned about your liver's role in filtering, trans-forming, and eliminating both internal (endo) and external (exo) toxins from your body. Chapter 2 offered an overview of the medical conditions that can result when your liver is burdened by those toxins. In this chapter, we'll take a look at just how this amazing organ processes every single thing we consume.

Your liver is like a screening station: It performs triage for your body, recognizing millions of potentially harmful chemicals and either trans-forming them into something harmless or preparing them for elimination. To accomplish this daunting task, it engages in a number of processes, including a two-phase detoxification procedure, as Leo Galland, MD, describes in *Power Healing.*[1] Let's begin with a brief over-view of both phases and then look more closely at each of them.

Phase One

In Phase One, your liver uses oxygen and enzymes (specifically, it uses the P450 family of enzymes) to burn toxins in a process called oxida-tion—a chemical process that adds oxygen to a particular compound and, in the process, eliminates one or more electrons.

Remember those many water- and fat-soluble toxins we learned about in Chapter 1—pesticides, preservatives, food additives, pollutants,

> **Compound:** A substance made up of two or more chemically bonded elements.
> **Electron:** A subatomic particle with a negative net charge.
> **Reactive Intermediate Toxins:** By-products from Phase One detoxification (such as free radicals), considered even more toxic than the original toxins.

plastics, and other environmental chemicals? Here in Phase One, your liver uses oxygen and enzymes to transform fat-soluble toxins into water-soluble ones so they can be eliminated from your body through your urine.

This first detoxification phase is critical. Remember, the only way fat-soluble toxins can exit your body is for them to be converted into water-soluble chemicals. But that poses risks, because while some toxins are either neutralized or reduced to a less toxic form and then eliminated from your body, others are changed into an even more toxic form. These toxins are often called "reactive intermediate toxins." Benzene—a dangerous solvent and carcinogen found in gasoline and cigarettes—is one example.[2] Enzymes in Phase One oxidize benzene, producing benzene quinones, which are even more toxic than the original substance.[3]

Phase Two

To get rid of toxins produced during its Phase One detoxification process, your liver must complete a second detox phase called conjugation. Here, conjugation refers to the combining of two compounds. In Phase Two, your liver combines specific nutrients to those reactive intermediate toxins produced by Phase One in order to render them harmless.

Let's take an in-depth look into your liver's two-phase detoxification process to see how food affects both detoxification and your overall health and well-being. We'll begin by looking back at a bit of history to see the connections scientists have made between what you eat and how well your body thrives.

Nutrition's Role in Detoxification: A Process of Discovery

Since the first vitamins and minerals were discovered in the early 1900s, followed by the discovery of enzymes in the 1930s, scientists have been trying to understand the role nutrition plays in our health and well-being. It's a complicated task. After all, when enzymes were first discovered, researchers could identify 80 of them. Now, less than a century later, scientists have identified more than 5,000 enzymes.[4] Two scientists in particular, Francis Pottenger, MD, and Weston Price, DDS, contributed significantly to our present understanding of how nutrition affects your liver's ability to detoxify your body.

The Cat Study

In 1930, physician and scientist Francis Pottenger performed a now-famous feeding experiment with cats that spanned more than 5 decades and many feline generations. His findings transformed the prevailing view of the role diet plays in health and well-being.

His experiment involved one group of cats who were fed varying degrees of denatured, processed foods and another group who were fed varying degrees of raw, fresh, high-quality, unprocessed foods. Over several generations, he observed the effects of the inferior diet. The cats who consumed the inferior, processed-food diet showed increased incidence of birth defects, stress-driven behaviors, vulnerability to illness, allergies, reduced learning capabilities, and significant reproductive problems. When Dr. Pottenger attempted to reverse the effects in the genetically weakened and vulnerable cats with a greatly improved diet, it took four generations for the cats to return to normal.[5]

Dr. Pottenger's work with cats revealed the connection between whole, fresh, high-quality foods and long-term health. In *Pottenger's Cats*, Dr. Pottenger applies his findings to humans. He explores the benefits of raw milk, nutrient-dense whole foods, and high-quality saturated fat to human health and well-being and shows the correlation between processed, denatured food and physical degeneration, including heart problems; liver, kidney, and bladder infections; thyroid dysfunction; and systemic inflammation. As your body's primary filter, when your liver is also burdened with the job of breaking down, transforming, and eliminating denatured, processed food, it's easy to see how health issues resulting from toxic overload can develop.

The Tooth Study

Dr. Weston Price, a dentist, lived from 1870 to 1948, when the first processed and industrialized foods were finding their way into our pantries and kitchens. Motivated by the death of his son from an infected tooth—and by his personal experience while eating mostly processed and industrialized foods—Dr. Price sought to determine how and why tooth decay occurs.

This question led him to study the effects these new foods had on people, compared to the effects of traditional foods. Dr. Price traveled the world, comparing those who were eating these new products (such as

{Agribusiness: *From Farm to Factory*

Industrial foods are produced on large factory farms, where thousands of animals are confined in massive warehouses and single crops are grown on thousands of acres. Agribusiness relies on the regular administration of drugs, hormones, and chemicals to keep the animals well and productive and on pesticides and on petroleum to produce abundant crops. The United Nations reports that factory farming is one of the top contributors to our planet's most significant environmental problems, including "land degradation, climate change, air pollution, water shortage, water pollution, and loss of biodiversity."[6]

processed cereals, canned foods, jams, white sugar, white flour, deli meats, and vegetable oils) to those who ate traditional, unprocessed whole foods. He observed 14 healthy groups of people living in various places, including the United States, the British Isles, Switzerland, Peru, and Africa, to name just a few. Each of the representative groups ate very different diets, yet they all exhibited some remarkable similarities.

In *Nutrition and Physical Degeneration,* he recounts several distinct patterns he discerned in all groups he studied. Two of the most important are:

- Those who ate newer foods—refined sugar, white flour, processed meats, and vegetable oils—had widespread tooth decay and little resistance to disease.

- Those who ate their country's traditional food were robust and healthy, with wide jaws to support good tooth structure. They suffered few, if any, cavities and exhibited a resistance to contemporary diseases, such as tuberculosis.[7]

Dr. Price documented pictures of people's teeth and facial structure, revealing the significant difference between those who ate traditional foods and those who didn't. Then he went on to analyze the nutrient content of the various foods participants were eating. Using dried food samples, he assessed specific nutrients in both the newer, processed foods and traditional, whole foods.

Despite varying countries and diets, Dr. Price discovered that traditional foods contained substantially higher amounts of minerals and vitamins than the refined and processed foods that were flooding the market at the time. He found that specific minerals and vitamins were significantly higher in traditional foods—for example, more calcium and vitamins A, D, and K_2 were found in butter made from milk from grass-fed cows.

Subsequently, Dr. Price began to treat underprivileged children who were sick and had severe tooth decay. For one meal a day, he fed them mineral-rich stews made of bone broths, plus raw milk, fresh vegetables, butter, fruit, cod liver oil, and whole wheat bread made with freshly ground wheat. A large percentage of these children began healing their cavities, though they were eating only one nutrient-dense meal each day.

With extensive documentation from six continents, Dr. Price concluded that a diet comprising whole, mineral-rich foods, including grass-fed animal fats, can provide continuing generations with healthy teeth, strong bone structure, and freedom from degenerative diseases.[8]

Since the middle of the 20th century, research like this has continued, showing that nutrient-dense foods improve the liver's two-phase detoxification process, improving overall health and well-being.[9]

Contemporary Voices

Today, many well-known physicians continue to assert that the foods we consume have a direct correlation to the health of the liver, and thus to our overall health and well-being. Among them:

Arthur Agatston, MD, author of *The South Beach Diet*
William Davis, MD, author of *Wheat Belly*
Michael Eades, MD, and Mary Dan Eades, MD, authors of *Protein Power*
Leo Galland, MD, author of *The Fat Resistance Diet*
Elson Haas, MD, author of *Staying Healthy with Nutrition*
Mark Hyman, MD, and Mark Liponis, MD, authors of *Ultraprevention*
Christiane Northrup, MD, author of *Women's Bodies, Women's Wisdom*
Andrew Perricone, MD, author of *The Perricone Prescription*
Michael Roizen, MD, and Mehmet Oz, MD, authors of *YOU: On a Diet*
Barry Sears, PhD, author of *The Zone Diet*
Andrew Weil, MD, author of *Spontaneous Healing*

Given your liver's formidable task of filtering, transforming, and eliminating everything that enters your body, it's easy to see how food has a significant impact on its ability to detox your body every 24 hours. The following section will explain exactly what effect food has on both phases of your liver's detoxification process.

Risky Business: Phase One

Phase One is crucial for detoxification. Many toxins—pesticides, preservatives, pollutants, plastics, heavy metals, and other environmental chemicals—would find their way into our fat stores without it. Yet, while it's essential, Phase One detoxification creates potential hazards.

Danger #1. Intermediate toxic compounds that aren't neutralized or eliminated create free radicals. These are molecules that are missing one or more electrons. These incomplete molecules create the kind of cell damage that can lead to cancer, degenerative diseases, and aging. As your liver works harder to detoxify your body, free radicals increase proportionally, as does inflammation. As free radicals increase, your body becomes vulnerable to long-term disease.

Danger #2. These reactive intermediate compounds are more toxic than the original substances. If your liver can't complete its Phase Two detox of these intermediate compounds, these toxins permeate your liver and infiltrate your entire body.

The research is vast and clear: Your food (and the nutrients or lack thereof in your food) plays a critical role in your liver's ability to filter, transform, and eliminate toxins, laying the foundation for (or sabotaging) your health and well-being. A group of nutrients that play a significant role in your liver's ability to detox your body are antioxidants.

Antioxidants and Detoxification

Since Phase One can produce unwanted free radicals and reactive intermediate toxins, your body needs antioxidants to further support the detoxification process. Antioxidants are natural micronutrients and your body's best protection against the damaging effects of free radicals.

(continued on page 56)

To support your liver's first detoxification phase, look for foods that help support your body's ability to create glutathione (GSH) levels, while supplying vitamins A, B$_1$, B$_2$, C, E, and zinc.[10] Here's a quick guide.

Vegetables

These vegetables provide substantial amounts of sulfur, vitamins, and antioxidants, which stimulate detox enzymes.

Cruciferous vegetables, such as broccoli, broccoli rabe, Brussels sprouts, cabbage, cauliflower, kale, turnip greens, watercress
Garlic

Lettuce, leaf and romaine
Mushrooms, shitake and reishi
Okra
Onions
Spinach

These vegetables also appear to boost GSH levels.

Acorn squash
Asparagus
Beets
Carrots
Cucumbers

Okra
Peppers, green bell
Peppers, sweet red
Sweet Potatoes
Zucchini

Fruits

These fruits help increase GSH levels.

Apples
Avocados
Berries
Cantaloupe
Grapes
Lemons
Limes

Mangos
Oranges
Papayas
Peaches
Pears
Tomatoes
Watermelon

These fruits are loaded with vitamin C, which stimulates GSH production while helping to bind and eliminate heavy metals such as mercury and cadmium.

Lemons
Limes

Oranges

These fruits provide significant amounts of antioxidants, vitamins, and minerals, all of which help maintain sufficient levels of GSH.

Apples	Melons
Avocados	Papayas
Berries	Peaches
Grapes	Pears
Mangos	Tomatoes

Animal- and Plant-Based Protein

Most sources of organic, grass-fed, free-range, or wild protein provide high levels of zinc, which helps boost glutathione levels. These include:

Beef	Fish
Chicken	Pork

If you're a vegan, you can support your liver well with vegetables, fruits, nuts and seeds (hemp seeds are particularly high in protein), plant-based fats, legumes, and grains, such as quinoa. As legumes and many grains require much work on the part of your digestive system, it's best to sprout these. More on this later (see page 99).

Organic Whey Protein

Whey protein is a great source of the amino acid cysteine and additional amino acids that are used for glutathione production. The benefits of dairy continue to be controversial, but many researchers believe that whey protein may be an exception, with a few conditions: The whey protein should be made from organic, cold-processed concentrate because cold processing not only boosts glutathione levels significantly, but also allows some of the beneficial bacteria to remain active. And ideally, the whey protein should be derived from organic, grass-fed cows that have not been exposed to pesticides, hormones, or antibiotics.

Spices

Several spices raise GSH levels, including:

Cardamom
Cinnamon
Curcumin (found in turmeric)

Free radicals are molecules that have lost an electron as a result of the natural process of oxidation. New cells are being created constantly, and old cells are always dying off. In the process, a small percentage of cells are damaged when oxygen interacts with their cellular tissue, in much the same way that vegetables and fruits spoil if left out on the counter for too long. This damage results in free radicals, which in turn go looking for their lost electron. It's easy to see how free radicals can wreak widespread destruction in your body without the help of antioxidants.

Here's how antioxidants work: They provide one or more of their extra electrons to free radicals, those toxins that are short one or more electrons. In donating an electron to free radicals, antioxidants neutralize free radicals and halt the oxidative stress in your cells. Just as there are two sources of toxins, there are also two main sources of antioxidants: exogenous and endogenous.

EXOGENOUS ANTIOXIDANTS.

Exo means "outside," so exogenous antioxidants are those you derive from your diet by eating colorful, nutrient-rich foods, spices, and herbs. Your liver needs these exogenous antioxidants for both Phase One and Phase Two detoxification. We'll learn more about food-based antioxidants later in this chapter (see pages 62 to 67).

ENDOGENOUS ANTIOXIDANTS

Endo means "inside," so endogenous antioxidants are made within your body. Because they're generated by your body and are not obtained from your food, endogenous antioxidants are equally, if not more, potent than exogenous antioxidants. They repair all of the free radical damage within your body by regenerating your cells from the inside out. Exogenous antioxidants, on the other hand, aren't quite so efficient. Instead of regenerating cells, they help promote cell renewal and growth in some (but not all) cells.

Five extremely powerful endogenous antioxidants reside in your body: glutathione (GSH), alpha lipoic acid (ALA), superoxide dismutase (SOD), catalase, and coenzyme Q_{10} (CoQ_{10}). We'll focus on glutathione, as it plays a crucial role in both the liver's Phase One and Phase Two detoxification.

Glutathione, an endogenous molecule derived from three amino acids—cysteine, glycine, and glutamine—is often considered to be the most important antioxidant for neutralizing the free radicals produced during Phase One. In fact, it may be one of your body's most important antioxidants, period. It transforms free radicals, detoxifies your body, protects your cells from oxidative stress, and strengthens your immune system.[10]

Glutathione is known by its abbreviation, GSH; the "SH" suffix indicates that the molecule contains the compound sulfhydryl. Your body obtains the sulfhydryl from the amino acids cysteine and methionine, both of which contain sulfur. In fact, the secret to glutathione's power may be in the sulfur it contains. Sulfur is a sticky, smelly molecule that acts like a sponge, drawing toxins in your body into itself, including free radicals and toxic compounds like mercury and heavy metals. Glutathione then transfers these toxins into bile and stool, to be eliminated from your body.

In *Glutathione: The Ultimate Antioxidant,* author Alan Pressman suggests that GSH is considered the master antioxidant because, unlike the others, it doesn't need additional antioxidants to do its job. Plus, with the most electrons to share, it's significantly stronger than any other antioxidant.[11]

Your liver needs significant amounts of GSH to detoxify your body, but those levels diminish in proportion to increasing levels of toxins in your body. Therefore, it's critical for you to maintain sufficient GSH levels.

Risky Business: Phase Two

In Phase Two, your liver transforms, neutralizes, or eliminates those reactive intermediate toxins from Phase One. While Phase One oxidizes toxins, Phase Two conjugates them, using sulfur and specific amino acids to convert oxidized chemicals into nontoxic compounds. In this phase, your liver can turn chemicals and toxins into substances your body can excrete.

{Phase Two Superfoods

Supporting Phase Two liver detox begins with food. Just as in Phase One, glutathione (GSH) plays a substantial role, so look to those foods that stimulate the production of specific enzymes, plus the glutathione conjugation needed during this second phase.

Cruciferous Vegetables
These foods speed up the production of the enzyme glutathione S-transferase and help it work better. This enzyme helps glutathione connect with toxins in order to neutralize them in Phase Two detoxification.

Bok choy	Cauliflower
Broccoli	Kale
Brussels sprouts	Scallions
Cabbage	

Allium Family Vegetables
The onion and its relatives, shallots, scallions, and leeks, contain sulfur compounds, which support the production of glutathione.

Leeks	Scallions
Onions	Shallots

Citrus Fruits
Lemons and limes contain high concentrations of vitamin C, which your body needs to make glutathione.

Lemons	Limes

Here's how the Phase Two conjugation process works: Your liver uses amino acids, enzymes, additional GSH, and particular nutrients (such as glutamine, choline, and inositol) to transform

Animal- and Plant-Based Protein

In addition to cruciferous vegetables, adequate protein intake appears to support Phase Two detoxification. Just as in Phase One, it's best to consider organic, grass-fed, free-range, or wild animal protein.

Beef	Pork
Chicken	Whey protein powder
Fish	

If you don't eat animal protein, choose vegetables, fruits, nuts and seeds (hemp seeds are great sources of protein), plant-based fats, legumes, and grains, such as quinoa. Legumes and grains can be difficult to digest, so sprouting is best (see page 99).

Spices—Curcumin

Curcumin, a phytochemical in the spice turmeric, a component of curry, is also beneficial in supporting your body's production of glutathione.

Sulfur-Based Amino Acids

Remember how your liver conjugates toxic compounds by using sulfur-based amino acids to neutralize those toxins? Three of these amino acids—cysteine, taurine, and methionine—play a critical role in Phase Two detoxification. The detoxification process depletes your body's storage of these amino acids. Thus the greater your toxic stress, the more your body demands these essential nutrients. To maintain your body's supply, eat sulfur-rich foods to continually replenish its stock.

Cruciferous vegetables	Meat
Eggs	Onions
Fish	Poultry
Garlic, raw	Shallots
Leeks	

Vegan sources of cysteine and methionine include:

Beans	Seeds
Nuts	

intermediate toxins into water-soluble substances that your body can easily excrete.

In water-soluble form, your body can excrete toxins via watery fluids, such as bile or urine. This is how your liver detoxifies some exotoxins, such as acetaminophen (Tylenol) and penicillin, as well as some endotoxins, such as hormones. During this second detox process, once again glutathione plays a key role.

Unfortunately, given the standard American diet and our stressful lifestyles, Phase Two detoxification may not be completed. Exposure to toxins, acetaminophen, alcohol, nutritional deficiencies, and low protein intake impede Phase Two by depleting essential enzymes, amino acids, and GSH levels—all of which your liver needs to complete this second phase. Let's take a look at how your diet and the environment can sabotage your liver's ability to complete its job.

Refined and processed foods, many vegetable oils, and charred meats, along with nitrates and preservatives, interrupt Phase Two detox. Caffeine, alcohol, smog, secondhand smoke, medications, hormone supplements (such as birth control pills and hormone replacement therapy), and excessive antibiotics further stress your liver. Regularly consuming many of these foods and chemicals can sabotage your liver's Phase Two process, causing toxins to accumulate in your body. These chemicals and toxins can erode your GSH levels more quickly than your diet can help produce them. If you have low levels of GSH, your body is more likely to experience oxidative stress, liver damage, and diseases like cancer that can be induced by toxins—especially if your Phase One detox system is highly active.[12]

In *Detoxify or Die*, Sherry Rogers, MD, notes that the cost of your liver's need for GSH in detoxification is high. For every toxic molecule you ingest, your body uses up a molecule of glutathione and magnesium. Each time your liver detoxifies a toxic chemical, you are requiring your body to supply energy and nutrients. This puts a huge demand on your body—day in and day out.[13]

Supporting Detox with Good Nutrition

As we've learned from earlier scientists, including Dr. Pottenger and Dr. Price, as well as a host of contemporary physicians and researchers, food is your body's fuel and medicine. It can either contribute to or diminish your health and well-being by either nourishing or sabotaging your liver's detoxification process. We've looked at specific foods that support Phase One and Phase Two detox individually. Now let's take a look at how some specific nutrients—alpha lipoic acid (ALA), selenium, antioxidants, carotenoids, and bioflavonoids, as well as their food sources—support both phases of your liver's detoxification process.

Alpha Lipoic Acid (ALA)

Alpha lipoic acid is a fatty acid found naturally inside every cell of your body. ALA converts blood glucose into energy, thus supplying your body with the necessary energy to perform routine functions. Alpha lipoic acid is also an antioxidant, neutralizing free radicals. It's unique among antioxidants because it can function both in water and oil or fat, unlike more common antioxidants, such as vitamins C and B, which function only in water.

Importantly, ALA appears to be able to recycle the antioxidants glutathione and vitamin C after they've been depleted. In addition, ALA increases the formation of glutathione.

Food sources of ALA are:

Broccoli	Spinach
Brussels sprouts	Tomatoes

Selenium

The antioxidant glutathione uses selenium to trap toxins and bind them to itself. Your body needs selenium to produce optimal levels of detoxifying glutathione-based enzymes.

Food sources of selenium are:

Brazil nuts	Oatmeal
Brewer's yeast	Onions
Brown rice	Salmon
Chicken	Seafood
Dairy products	Tuna
Eggs	Vegetables (most)
Garlic	Wheat germ
Molasses	Whole grains

Antioxidants, Vitamins and Minerals

Antioxidants, plus several minerals, are your best protection against the free-radical damage that results from the detoxification process. Minerals play a significant role in forming blood, bones, and teeth, as well as regulating body fluids. You need a robust supply of antioxidants and minerals, present in bright, deep-colored vegetables and fruits, herbs, and spices.

For Phase One, you need the antioxidant glutathione, along with vitamins A, B_1, B_2, C, and E, plus zinc.

For Phase Two, you need glutathione, folic acid (a vitamin in B complex), vitamin E, and the minerals selenium and manganese.

To limit free radical–induced damage, your body employs a defense system of protective enzymes and circulating antioxidants. Those antioxidants, which must come from food, include vitamin C, vitamin E, vitamin A, carotenoids and related bioflavonoids, along with the minerals selenium, manganese, copper, zinc, and sulfur (which is usually consumed as part of protein).

Vitamin C–Rich Foods. These include:

Berries
Cantaloupe
Dark green vegetables
  (asparagus, broccoli,
  Brussels sprouts, green bell
  peppers, spinach, and
  watercress and other
  greens)

Fruits, citrus (and their juices)
Guava
Mangos
Papaya
Pineapple
Red and yellow peppers
Tomatoes

Vitamin E–Rich Foods. These include:

Brown rice
Dark leafy green vegetables
Legumes (beans, lentils, split
  peas)
Nuts and nut butters

Oatmeal
Olive and safflower oils
Seeds
Sweet potatoes

Vitamin A–Rich Foods. These include:

Carrots
Cayenne, chile, and red pepper
Dark leafy greens

Sweet potatoes
Winter squashes (such as
  butternut and acorn)

Carotenoids and Bioflavonoids. Carotenoids and bioflavonoids are potent antioxidants that are found in many colorful fruits and vegetables. These antioxidants offer protection against free radicals and oxidative stress, both of which can lead to inflammatory diseases such as cancer, atherosclerosis, and autoimmune conditions.

Carotenoids. These are a type of natural pigment that give dark orange, red, yellow, and green vegetables and fruits their colors. Carotenoids help your body produce retinol, a form of vitamin A. The primary carotenoid is beta-carotene, the orange pigment evident in carrots and cantaloupe. Foods rich in carotenoids include:

Apricots

Broccoli

Cantaloupe

Carrots

Collards

Dandelion greens

Kale

Mustard greens

Papaya

Pumpkin

Red peppers

Spinach

Sea vegetables (dulse, hiziki,
    kelp, nori, and wakame)

Sweet potatoes

Swiss chard

Tomatoes

Winter squash

Bioflavonoids. Found in many plants, bioflavonoids are natural compounds that supply a range of colors in many fruits, vegetables, and spices, ranging from bright yellow in curcumin (a phytonutrient in turmeric curry) and ginger to deep purple in Concord grapes. Bioflavonoids are powerful antioxidants that may help:

- Neutralize free radicals

- Suppress inflammation and allergic reactions by decreasing production of natural chemicals by immune cells

- Protect your body against cancer by preventing division of malignant cells

- Protect your cardiovascular system from damage by toxins and other harmful chemicals

- Keep your blood cholesterol at healthy levels, protecting your blood vessels from atherosclerosis

Foods rich in bioflavonoids include:

Asparagus, green tips only

Beets

Black cherries

Blackberries

Blueberries

Cranberries

Ginger

Milk thistle (herb)

Purple corn

Purple onions

Radishes

Rhubarb

Red cabbage

Sweet potatoes

Red grapes

Turmeric

Raspberries

Folic Acid Derived from Folate-Rich Foods. Folic acid is a vitamin B that the body derives from folate-rich foods. Folic acid helps your body form red blood cells and helps protect them from atherosclerosis. Foods rich in folates are:

Beets

Dark leafy greens

Broccoli

Legumes

Cauliflower

Zinc-Rich Foods. Zinc, an important antioxidant used in Phase One detox, is found in:

Beans

Pumpkin seeds

Dairy products

Red meat

Nuts

Seafood

Oysters

Whole grains

Poultry

Selenium-Rich Foods. Selenium plays a critical role in both creating glutathione and breaking down toxins in your liver. Selenium is

Superflavonoids

Some flavonoids are super effective. Turmeric is found in curry powder and has traditionally been used to treat arthritis and inflammation. Ginger, which contains more than 400 chemically active ingredients, has long been used to relieve digestive complaints and motion sickness and to aid circulation. Milk thistle is a longtime herbal treatment for the liver. The active ingredients are a group of bioflavonoids collectively called silymarin. Research indicates that milk thistle may offer protection from liver disease.[14]

{The Antioxidant Top 20

Support your local liver! Eat some of these foods daily. For quick reference, here's a list of the top 20 best food sources of antioxidants, as measured by the total antioxidant capacity per serving size.[15] Notice that these foods are all plant based, providing a significant amount of powerful micronutrients that restore, renew, and regenerate cells throughout your body.

ANTIOXIDANT	SERVING SIZE	TOTAL ANTIOXIDANT CAPACITY PER SERVING
1. Small Red Beans	½ cup	13,727
2. Wild blueberries	1 cup	13,427
3. Red kidney beans	½ cup	13,259
4. Pinto beans	½ cup	11,864
5. Blueberries (cultivated)	1 cup	9,019
6. Cranberries	1 cup	8,983
7. Artichoke Hearts	1 cup	7,904
8. Blackberries	1 cup	7,701
9. Prunes	½ cup	7,291
10. Raspberries	1 cup	6,058
11. Strawberries	1 cup	5,938
12. Red delicious apples	1	5,900
13. Granny Smith apples	1	5,381
14. Pecans	1 ounce	5,095
15. Sweet cherries	1 cup	4,873
16. Black plums	1	4,844
17. Russet potatoes, cooked	1	4,649
18. Black beans	½ cup	4,181
19. Plums	1	4,118
20. Gala apples	1	3,903

abundant in small fish, like sardines and anchovies, as well as chicken and turkey. It's also present in some herbs and spices—curry powder, turmeric, and milk thistle.

Manganese-Rich Foods. These foods are rich in manganese:

Dark leafy greens	Whole grains, such as brown
Garbanzo beans	rice, oats, and spelt
Pumpkin seeds	

While many of these foods are beneficial, some are not recommended on the cleanse. Legumes, for example, challenge your digestive system, and the cleanse aims to reduce its work on incoming foods, so it can clean itself of digested matter. White potatoes and sweeter fruits are not recommended because of their carbohydrates and sugar. Postcleansing, these are beautiful antioxidants to consume.

The Bottom Line

The only way your body can complete Phase Two is with a robust liver. And for that to happen, it's a simple formula: The rate at which Phase One produces activated intermediate toxins must be balanced by the rate at which Phase Two can finish their processing.

Unfortunately for many of us, because of our overconsumption of exotoxins and our production of endotoxins, our livers often can't accomplish this second phase. And when that happens, your body becomes overloaded with additional toxins that eventually make their way back to your liver, contributing to fluid retention, weight gain, and the wide array of health issues we looked at in Chapter 2.

The importance of a clean and healthy liver can't be overstated. It supports your body in digesting and assimilating the nutrients in your food, metabolizing fat, and flushing your system of both toxins and free radicals. All these essential processes lead to increased energy, vitality, and balance. Plus, a well-functioning liver helps you obtain the maximum benefit from the foods you eat, letting you feel fuller and more satisfied both earlier and longer.

Now that you understand how essential your liver is, what an arduous job it performs with every bite and breath you take, what happens when it's overburdened, how you feel when it can't complete its detoxifying process, and how specific foods either support or sabotage its efforts, it's easy to see why performing a liver cleanse is so critical to your overall health and well-being. Before we jump into the process, we need to clean, support, and nourish your entire digestive tract so that it can do its job of absorbing and assimilating critical nutrients while excreting toxins efficiently and effectively. In the next chapter, we'll learn how to heal and strengthen your digestive tract.

VANESSA CLARKE, 53

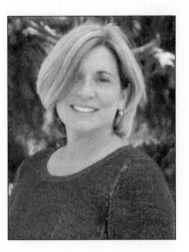

Organized at Last!

Clothes: Fit better

Energy levels: Way up

Piles of paperwork: Organized at last

I have three kids and I do a lot of volunteer work—last year I was head of the parents' fund at my children's private high school, and I was the corresponding secretary, Web designer, and digital correspondence secretary for an organization that benefits underprivileged children. It seemed like I had little piles of paperwork all over the house—little tasks that I could never get to and that always nagged at the back of my mind.

Well, that all changed while on the LiverUp! Cleanse. I wasn't sure I'd have the willpower to make it through, but I knew detoxes are good for you, and I just wanted to feel healthier and stronger. The first 3 days were tough, but once I got through them, it was just amazing. I had this overwhelming feeling of clarity and energy, and I even started sleeping better. I felt like Superwoman! I was more productive, and I even had time to organize my entire home. And all that paperwork? All those little piles that were just waiting for me to make a decision about them? Well, suddenly it all seemed so much easier. My mind was so clear that I could make those decisions in no time flat. For me, that was the biggest benefit of the cleanse.

But there were other benefits, too. I didn't do it to lose weight, but by the end of the cleanse my pants fit better and my stomach felt flatter. And it was wonderful to really enjoy food again. All my cravings for sugar and caffeine disappeared, and it seemed like my palate was rebooted. I remember eating a tomato and tasting the sweetness—everything tastes so good when you don't eat processed foods.

The whole experience gave me a sense of confidence and discipline over my eating. I learned a surprising lesson: It's healthy to be hungry. It just means your body is working properly. I'd thought that limiting my diet would make me feel deprived, but it wasn't like that at all. It gave me an amazing appreciation for food, and it showed me that I was surrounded by abundance.

CHAPTER 4

Healing Your Gut, Cleansing Your Colon

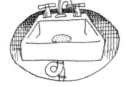

First things first: To free your body of stored toxins, you have to heal your gut and clean your colon. Your gut—your intestinal nervous system—is located in sheaths of tissue lining almost your entire digestive tract, which includes your esophagus, stomach, small intestine, and colon. In this chapter, we'll look at how your gut and colon play a significant role in detoxing your body, supporting your immune system, and boosting your overall health and well-being. Your entire digestive system is closely attuned to not only your physical health, but your emotional health, as well. Researchers at Swinburne University of Technology in Australia, for instance, found that during their final exams, the stool samples of stressed-out students contained fewer beneficial gut bacteria than they did during happier days at the start of the semester.[1]

And your liver is the key to your digestive health. Think of your digestive system as your kitchen plumbing: Your liver is the sieve, your gut is the sink, and your colon is the main drainage pipe. If your sink is dirty and your drainage pipe is clogged, toxins can permeate your entire body and make you sick.

Remember how your liver creates more than a quart of bile each day? How it carries toxic substances and dumps them into your intestines to be excreted? And on the way down the GI tract, how bile helps emulsify the fats you eat to help your small intestine digest and absorb

71

them? That's important: You need to be able to digest clean, healthy fats, which are essential for many of your body's processes—including those performed by your cardiovascular, reproductive, immune, and central nervous systems. In an amazing, continuous loop, these same bile salts are recycled from your intestines and back to your liver to do their job all over again—as many as 20 times.

This remarkable recycling system works beautifully if your entire digestive system is in good order. When your gut is healthy and your colon is working smoothly, your body is absorbing nutrients and expelling waste efficiently and effectively.

But if your gut is distressed or your colon is congested, that loop is compromised. Congested intestines wreak havoc on your health, preventing the absorption and assimilation of essential nutrients, allowing food to putrefy in your colon and toxins to seep into your body, and inhibiting the recirculation of bile salts back to your liver, which slows down bile production.

Bile is essential, both in metabolizing fats and stimulating peristalsis, the muscular movement that propels food along your digestive tract. So low bile levels can lead to constipation as toxins, bile, and greasy, undigested fats sit in your intestines for too long. If this matter lingers long enough, it hardens and causes your intestines to expand, adding weight and inches to your abdomen.

If these toxins aren't eliminated, your body will eventually reabsorb them and send them back to your liver all over again. So when your intestines are sluggish, toxins, bile, and undigested fats accumulate in your colon, impairing not only your digestive process, but also your liver's detoxification process. The consequences? Many of the symptoms we learned about in Chapter 2.

So where do we begin to set things right? One of the first steps in detoxing your liver—and thus your entire body—is to clear and flush downstream before you scour upstream, so that the toxins your liver has released can exit your body effectively and efficiently through your intestines and colon. When your GI tract is clogged, those toxins travel back up to your liver and get stored in your tissues.

Let's take a look downstream at your intestinal tract.

Gut Check

Your gut is made up of your stomach, intestines, and colon, and it's home to trillions of microorganisms, which should primarily be found in your colon. These gut bacteria coexist in an amazing, harmonious ecosystem. How many are there? Let's just say that you have way more bacteria in your gut than you have cells in your entire body.

Besides being well populated, your gut is also a very busy place. It's the principal area in your body where:

- Foreign matter is introduced, mainly through your mouth.

- Exchanges are made between you and the exterior world—in at the top and out at the bottom.

- Nutrients are absorbed by your body, mainly in your small intestine, with additional work by your teeth and mouth, salivary glands, stomach, stomach acid and enzymes, pancreas, and of course your liver and its hardworking bile.

Your gut bacteria, often called gut flora, are vital organisms, literally. Without them, you wouldn't survive. Scientists are constantly learning new ways that digestive health and the health of your gut flora are linked to the health of your entire body—your gut flora plays an important part in the function of your immune system, the way you digest your food, how you absorb nutrients and produce energy, and much more.[2] This is so significant that the FDA has approved fecal transplants, a procedure where probiotic-rich feces are taken from one person and placed in another. For those suffering with debilitating intestinal health problems, the procedure has proven to be life changing.[3]

Since your gut is the major system that comes into contact with toxins and pathogens, it's where most diseases begin. And that's why it's imperative that you take care of your intestinal flora—abnormal or damaged gut flora is one of the root causes of all disease, as scientists are learning all the time. A team of researchers at Freiburg University in Germany infected two groups of mice—one that had normal intestinal flora and another that had no intestinal flora at all—with viruses. Those with the healthy, normal gut flora were able to fight off the viruses, while those without gut flora became ill. But when scientists provided the second group of mice with gut flora, their immune response improved.[4] Scientists, continuing to study these questions in humans, believe that by caring for your gut flora you may prevent or even reverse conditions including heart disease, autoimmune diseases, allergies, and even cancer.[5]

Balancing Act

Your intestinal flora consists of trillions of "friendly" and "unfriendly" microorganisms, all coexisting in a communal, symbiotic relationship. These microorganisms, which inhabit the various regions of your digestive tract, make up nearly 4 pounds of your total body weight. And the way they're balanced—ideally, 85 percent "friendly" bacteria to 15 percent "unfriendly"—affects how healthy you are and how vibrant you feel.[6] Here are some of the essential jobs these microorganisms do.

- They protect against pathogens, viruses, harmful bacteria, and yeast. Friendly bacteria, also known as probiotics, slow the multiplication of many dangerous pathogens, particularly fungi, by competing with and replacing them on your intestinal walls.[7]

- They stimulate the function of your entire digestive system, keeping it moving.

- They help balance optimum pH levels in your colon. A healthy alkalinity-to-acidity ratio boosts your immune response and inhibits the growth of fungus and mycotoxin (fungal poison) production.[8]

- They prevent inflammation in your gut and throughout your entire body.[9]

- They support proper metabolism and weight regulation.

- They help your body maintain high energy levels by detoxifying your colon, kidneys, and liver.

- They help counteract cancer-causing compounds in your colon.

But when the natural balance of your gastrointestinal tract is disturbed, your beneficial flora can't flourish, and toxin-producing bacteria and fungi begin to take over. When bad bacteria overpopulate your gut, it can lead to serious health problems. Among the better-known gut problems are inflammatory bowel disease (IBD), irritable bowel syndrome (IBS), gastroesophageal reflux disease (GERD), and celiac disease. Too many bad gut bacteria can even lead to problems outside your gut. Researchers at the Mayo Clinic and the University of Illinois at Urbana-Champaign, using mice genetically engineered with the human gene responsible for a predisposition to rheumatoid arthritis, showed that gut flora may contribute to a person's susceptibility to arthritis. Other systemic conditions, such as autoimmune diseases, are thought to stem from imbalances in and damage to the gut, as well. Inflammation in your gut may lead to inflammation in your joints or arteries, causing arthritis and atherosclerosis.[10]

Let's see how your gut flora either enhance or sabotage your health.

Beneficial "Friendly" Bacteria

Since your gut is the major organ that comes into contact with toxins and pathogens, it's headquarters for much of your immune system and digestive enzyme production. It's the foremost immune area in your body. Adequate levels of friendly bacteria (85 percent) to pathogenic "unfriendly" bacteria (15 percent) prevent harmful, toxin-producing fungi from taking over your gastrointestinal tract, suppressing your immune cells and their response.[11] The most beneficial bacteria:

- Bifidobacteria (*Bifidobacterium bifidum*)
- Lactobacteria (*Lactobacillus acidophilus*, *L. plantarum*, and *L. rhamnosus*)

Beneficial bacteria create a natural barrier called the *mucosal barrier,* to protect your body against invading bacteria, parasites, fungi, viruses, and toxins that reside in most everything you eat and drink. They also reduce acidity levels near the wall of your gut so that unfriendly bacteria can't live there.

Opportunistic "Unfriendly" Bacteria

Unfriendly bacteria live right alongside friendly bacteria in your gut. Among them are:

- Bacilli
- Bacteroides
- Parasites

- Staphylococci
- Streptococci
- Yeasts

So far, scientists have identified about 500 species of microbes in the intestinal tract. When you're healthy, those friendly bacteria keep the unfriendly ones down to size. That's because each of these "bad" microbes can cause health problems when they overpopulate.[12] So it's critical to maintain a healthy ratio of friendly to unfriendly bacteria in your GI tract. Without the right balance, these bad bacteria and fungi can overproduce and trigger a host of health concerns.

Intermediary, Transitional Bacteria

Intermediary or transitional bacteria include a variety of microbes you consume every day in what you eat and drink. When your gut is healthy, with the right ratio of beneficial bacteria, that's no problem. Those microbes zip along your digestive tract without causing any trouble. But if your population of beneficial flora is damaged or isn't working quite right because of antibiotics, birth control pills, hormone treatments, steroidal treatments, fluoride, chlorine, carbonated drinks, radiation, preservatives, additives, pesticides, fertilizers, environmental toxins, heavy metals, or excess sugar and processed carbohydrates—on top of excessive stress—these microbes can cause disease.[13]

Your Beneficial Flora at Work

In your gut, beneficial flora are responsible for very important functions, from helping your body digest and assimilate your food to strengthening your immune system. As almost all of your body's immune system lives in your gut (some experts say 90 percent), let's take a closer look at how your gut flora supports it.

Many researchers believe that nearly all disease can be traced back to the GI tract and digestive dysfunction, abnormal or damaged microbes, or inflammation.[14] That's why beneficial flora plays such a crucial role in supporting your immune system.

Much like your Phase One and Phase Two liver detoxification processes, your gut flora maintains two efforts of your immune system, keeping it in balance and encouraging it to respond appropriately to unfriendly microbes. Here's how these two efforts work.

First, your gut flora responds to all the toxins and chemicals you ingest—in the air you breathe, the food you eat, and the beverages you drink. Substances in the air (such as exhaust fumes, pollution, dust, pollen, animal dander), plus chemicals in your food, settle on your mucous membranes and travel farther into your gut.

When you have too few good gut flora, or when they're underfunctioning or damaged, unfriendly or "bad" bacteria can take up residence more readily and seep through your gut wall and into your body in a condition called leaky gut syndrome. When this happens, opportunistic bacteria, left unchecked by friendly bacteria, can weaken the integrity of your intestinal wall, allowing harmful substances that normally wouldn't pass through to seep out into your body. "Bad" microbes attach themselves to your gut lining, digging "roots" into the mucosal membranes and making it "leaky." That means that larger holes in the wall allow bigger molecules to be absorbed through it. Partially digested foods seep through this leaky gut wall and into your bloodstream. Other disease-causing microbes, plus a variety of toxins, can also enter through the leaky gut.

The second effort of your immune system kicks in when your "leaky gut" allows incompletely digested proteins to enter your bloodstream. As soon as it detects these foreign or unfamiliar particles, your immune system manufactures antibodies against them. The problem, however, is that some of those proteins mimic proteins already present in your body, so your immune system goes into overdrive, forming new antibodies to attack proteins that are almost identical to those already there.

Your body responds in an allergic or reactive way, with symptoms of conditions similar to asthma, hay fever, and allergies to dust, animals, food, and so on. Additional symptoms of leaky gut syndrome are:

- Bloating
- Fatigue
- Foggy thinking
- Intestinal cramps
- Mood swings
- Weak immunity
- Yeast overgrowth (candida)

If left untreated, leaky gut can lead to chronic immune hyperactivity—the root cause of autoimmune diseases such as celiac disease, multiple sclerosis (MS), Graves' disease, and rheumatoid arthritis (RA).[15] That makes healing your leaky gut even more important.

When Good Bacteria Go Bad

When your gut ecology gets disrupted, colonies of harmful, putrefying bacteria can discharge highly toxic by-products that react with foods in your digestive tract. This reaction can further upset your gastrointestinal tract, slowly poisoning your whole body and initiating the onset of chronic degenerative diseases, according to Heidi Nelson, MD, director of the Mayo Clinic's Microbiome Program.[16]

How does that happen? There are many culprits: Our environment, our lifestyles, and our food can all damage or undermine beneficial gut flora. Antibiotics such as penicillin and tetracycline can sabotage beneficial bacteria as well, not only in your gut, but in other organs and tissues, as well. Other dangers to your friendly bacteria are oral contraceptives, prolonged stress, exposure to toxic substances, and a poor diet. Foods and additives that can damage or stress your friendly bacteria include processed foods, chemicals, preservatives, and refined sugars and carbohydrates, as well as meat that comes from animals that are routinely injected with antibiotics, steroids, and other drugs. These foods create imbalance in your gut flora by producing a habitat in which "bad" bacteria thrive. And once things have gone awry, it takes between 4 and 8 weeks—depending on the species of beneficial bacteria—to reestablish those good bacteria in your gut.

As your beneficial flora fall prey to antibiotics, environmental toxins, and stress from your diet and lifestyle, there's a window of opportunity for disease-causing bacteria, viruses, and fungi to establish themselves along your intestinal walls. Your body can't thrive without well-functioning gut flora, so it's essential that you take care of your

Top 8 Bacteria Disrupters}

- Sugar
- Refined carbohydrates
- A diet rich in red meats and unhealthy fats
- Excessive carbonated cola and alcohol
- Processed foods
- Antibiotics
- Anti-inflammatory drugs and painkillers
- Stress

gut—it holds the keys to your health. The good news is that you can heal your gut and rebuild your friendly bacteria colonies with the foods on the LiverUp! Cleanse. Keep reading.

Healing Your Gut: The LiverUp! Cleanse

Given our standard American diet and stressful lives, most of us don't have the right levels of beneficial flora, which results in a compromised digestive system. To flush toxins out of your body with a liver cleanse, you need to heal your gut first.

The LiverUp! Cleanse begins with these three gut-healing principles: weeding, feeding, and seeding your digestive system. Here's what each phase of the cleanse will accomplish.

Weeding

You'll be clearing out those foods and chemicals that stress your gut and are toxic to your body.

- Conventionally raised animal proteins (including dairy), which may contain hormones, antibiotics, pesticides, herbicides, or heavy metals

- Processed foods that contain refined flour and little or no fiber

- Refined sugar

- Alcohol

- Soft drinks

- Partially hydrogenated fats

- Prepackaged foods that contain chemicals, dyes, or preservatives

Seeding

You'll be supporting your gut with foods rich in probiotics, beneficial microflora that support the health of your intestinal tract. Probiotics are microorganisms that mimic and strengthen the beneficial microorganisms living in your gut.

We humans have been eating probiotics in the form of fermented foods for thousands of years. Nobel Prize winner Élie Metchnikoff, a Russian physiologist, first hypothesized that consuming lactic acid–producing bacteria found in cultured dairy could be beneficial for health and longevity. He studied Bulgarian peasants who lived much longer than their European counterparts and came to believe that their longevity was due in large part to the raw, unprocessed, unpasteurized, fermented dairy drink they consumed daily. He theorized that the good bacteria in the "sour milk" they drank were responsible for balancing the bad bacteria in the gut. Metchnikoff isolated one species of probiotic (*Lactobacillus bulgaricus*) from cultured dairy. Today, many people are familiar with probiotics and the theory that these bacteria are significant in healing and supporting your gut, and thus your whole body. Metchnikoff is known as the "Father of Probiotics."[17]

Probiotics provide an array of health benefits, from helping with digestive disorders to boosting your immune system. They make your gastrointestinal system work more efficiently and boost your resistance to disease. Studies have shown that probiotics support your health and well-being by helping to:

- Digest nutrients[18]

- Alleviate common digestive disorders such as constipation, diarrhea, and IBS[19]

- Prevent and treat colon inflammation[20]

- Reduce incidence of yeast infections, including candida[21]

- Reduce bad breath

- Strengthen your immune system[22]

- Counteract negative side effects of antibiotics[23]

- Increase your body's ability to synthesize vitamin B and absorb calcium[24]

Feeding

You'll be feeding your gut with prebiotics, digestive enzymes, and hydrochloric acid (HCl) to stimulate the growth of intestinal flora. Prebiotics are indigestible fibers in food that help the probiotics in your intestines to flourish and grow. Prebiotics, unlike probiotics, aren't living organisms. They include oligofructose and inulin (naturally found in chicory root, onions, leeks, whole grains, and bananas). These fibers make their way to your digestive tract intact, serving as "growth hormones" for health-preserving bowel flora.[25]

In addition to prebiotics, digestive enzymes and hydrochloric acid (HCl) also help support your intestinal tract. Inadequate stomach acid and low pancreatic enzymes are both extremely common; they cause poor digestion and malabsorption. Typical symptoms of low stomach acid are the four Bs: burping, belching, burning, and bloating.

{Probiotic Superfoods

- Sauerkraut
- Microalgae
- Miso
- Tempeh
- Kimchi
- Yogurt (if you choose to eat dairy)
- Kefir (if you choose to eat dairy)
- Kombucha tea

Nausea and even acid reflux can be caused by a deficiency of HCl in your stomach. (Avoid betaine HCl if you have a peptic or duodenal ulcer or if you've had one in the past.)

So how exactly will you be feeding your gut during the cleanse? You'll be turning to these immune-supporting foods.

- Large amounts of fresh fruits and vegetables, particularly glutamine-rich foods, such as dandelion greens, parsley, Brussels sprouts, celery, spinach, and carrots. Glutamine is the main fuel source for millions of immune cells and those cells lining your intestines.

- Nuts and seeds

- Fish

- Bitter foods, such as radicchio, endive, and beet leaves

- Sour foods, such as lemon and lime

- Vegetable juices

- Milk thistle supplements

- Vitamin C

- Garlic

Choosing Foods Rich in Beneficial Bacteria and Probiotics

Here are a few probiotic-rich foods you should add to your diet. Whenever you can, opt for organic versions.

Sauerkraut. Sauerkraut, made from fermented cabbage and other vegetables, is loaded with healthy live cultures. It's also a great source of vitamins B, A, E, and C. (Try the delicious, simple recipe on page 260.)

Microalgae. Microalgae are superfood freshwater plants that include spirulina, chlorella, and blue-green algae. These foods are high in chlorophyll, a powerful detoxifier that can help you:

- Process more oxygen throughout your body, thus increasing your energy levels

- Support your key elimination systems—your bowel, liver, and blood

- Purify your blood and clean away toxins

- Promote growth and repair of your tissues

- Boost your immune system by increasing antioxidants and reducing inflammation

- Manage diabetes

- Improve your digestion

- Balance your body's pH

While the United States has been a bit slower to turn to these remarkable foods, some research findings have confirmed what the Japanese have known for years. In a study at the University of California, Davis, scientists enrolled 40 volunteers who were at least 50 years old and who had no history of major chronic diseases. They were given a spirulina supplement for 12 weeks and were administered comprehensive dietary questionnaires to determine their nutritional regimen during the study. Signs of immune function, complete cell count, and enzyme activity were determined at baseline and after weeks 6 and 12 of supplementation. Over the 12-week period, participants showed a steady increase in both cell count and enzyme activity, leading researchers to conclude that spirulina increases immune function by reducing inflammation and increasing antioxidant effects.[26]

A Korean study confirmed that spirulina helps manage type 2 diabetes. Patients with type 2 diabetes received spirulina or a placebo for 12 weeks. Those whose diets were supplemented with spirulina were found to have significantly reduced oxidative markers, such as triglycerides (fat in the blood), LDL cholesterol, inflammation, and blood pressure.[27]

Finally, a Medical College of Virginia study concluded that chlorella provides nutrients that can help resist infection and improve your immunity. Chlorella was used to treat 20 brain tumor patients whose immune systems were compromised after surgery, radiation, or chemotherapy. Over the 2-year study, researchers observed that these patients had fewer respiratory infections and flulike illnesses than usual for patients with these types of tumors. Seven patients remained alive, with no reappearance of their tumors after 2 years.[28]

Microalgae are among the most nutritious foods available anywhere.[29] They contain these fundamental nutrients.

- Amino acids, which provide the basic building blocks for all of life (spirulina contains 65 percent protein, more than any other natural food)

- Antioxidants (especially beta-carotene), which neutralize free radicals

- Vitamin B_{12} and B complex, absorbable iron, and essential trace minerals

- Essential fatty acids—particularly GLA, precursor to the body's prostaglandins (master hormones that control many functions)—EFAs provide structural components for cell membranes and play a critical role in brain and hormone chemistry

Miso. Miso, loaded with nutrients, is made from fermented soy, as well as rye, beans, rice, or barley. It's used widely in traditional Japanese medicine and macrobiotic cooking to support the digestive system. One tablespoon of miso in a cup of hot water makes a quick, delicious, and probiotic-rich soup that's full of lactobacilli and bifidobacteria.

Tempeh. A great substitute for meat or tofu, tempeh is a fermented soybean product that's rich in probiotics. Because it's fermented with bacteria, it's one of the few vegetarian sources that provides vitamin B_{12}.

(Spirulina and chlorella are others). This versatile, low-salt protein can be sautéed or baked and used in vegetable stir-fries or tossed into salads.

Kimchi. Kimchi is a spicy and sour Asian version of pickled sauerkraut, often served as a side dish. It's a rich source of calcium, iron, beta-carotene, and vitamins A and C, among many other important nutrients. See page 261 for a recipe for homemade kimchi, or you can buy it at most health food and grocery stores. Try to find varieties with no added coloring or preservatives.

Yogurt. Yogurt containing live cultures—especially homemade—is an excellent probiotic food if you choose to eat dairy. Your best bet? Yogurt made from goat's milk with added probiotics such as *Lactobacillus acidophilus*. Check the label before buying—avoid brands that contain high-fructose corn syrup, artificial flavorings, or sweeteners.

Kefir. Kefir—a fermented dairy product made with milk and grains—is another great probiotic if you choose to eat dairy. It's loaded with the bacteria lactobacilli and bifidobacteria, as well as antioxidants. As always, organic is best.

Kombucha Tea. A healthy alternative to your morning cup of coffee, this fermented tea is a natural energy booster with lots of healthy probiotic bacteria. Avoid it, though, if you've had problems with candida yeast infections in the past.

What's Next?

Now that you understand the critical role your liver and gut play in your overall health and well-being, you're ready to take on the 12-day cleanse, which is designed to promote your healing in two ways.

1. It will clear your body of toxins that you've been storing for years.

2. It will support your body's major detox organs—your liver and colon—so they can continue to filter and eliminate toxins, allowing you to absorb life-giving nutrients.

During your 2-week cleanse, you'll add foods that support both Phase One and Phase Two detoxification and help your beneficial gut flora to thrive—all while forgoing those foods that sabotage the detoxification process and your gut flora. In short, you will eat foods that help:

- Nourish you with healthy nutrition

- Boost your glutathione levels

- Increase bile production

- Sweep clean your intestines

- Support your "friendly" bacteria

- Increase your supply of antioxidants

- Reduce your overall toxic load

During the cleanse, you'll be guided gently through the entire process and offered a variety of foods from which to choose for every meal. In addition, you'll find sample menus and recipes that help you detoxify your liver, plus daily exercises to flush out the toxins while calming your mind. You'll be encouraged to journal through the process, as a means to observe—with no judgment—the feelings, thoughts, emotions, and physical sensations you experience during this time.

As written in *The Yoga Sutras of Patanjali*—the classical text from the yoga school of Indian philosophy, written in the 2nd century BC— "Now is the time."[30] There was a reason you picked up this book. Now is the time for you to commit to detoxing and supporting your liver. It could change your life. Let's do it now.

JILL DANLY, 54

A Design for Health

Coffee addiction: Conquered

Concentration and thinking: Sharper

Energy levels: Better than ever

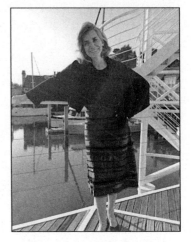

I'm an architect. I specialize in designing contemporary houses, but I also teach third-year architecture students at a university in Chicago. My teaching schedule can be demanding, with 5 hours of intense critique and conversation required, without a break.

For me, being on the cleanse makes everything seem so much sharper, so much more in focus, with nothing fogging my patterns of thought. The way I feel reminds me of a beautifully crafted architectural drawing that's made with precision and a clear idea of where the design is going.

I don't drink coffee before I go into class—that's definitely not the stimulant I need. I've learned from doing the cleanse that my stimulant should be the way I live my life and the clarity my food and my lifestyle provide. That's what allows me to get through those 5 hours while just drinking water and green tea, and maybe eating a handful of nuts. If it hadn't been for the cleanse and everything I learned from it, I think I'd still be having a lot of coffee!

I have repeated the cleanse on several occasions, and I've enjoyed it each time. I usually follow the suggestions and almost never waiver. The recipes are wonderful and making them is an experience in mindfulness. It's meditative on all levels. The cleanse jump-starts my healthful living. I'm left with such clarity and energy, and a complete sense of well-being.

CHAPTER 5

The 12-Day LiverUp! Cleanse

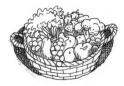

To flush your body of harmful toxins, food is the best medicine. You'll be amazed by how many delicious foods clean your detoxification organs—your liver, intestines, kidneys, lungs, and skin. Clean, whole foods help your liver and colon remove toxic buildup and ward off the harmful effects of pollution, food additives, secondhand smoke, and other toxins. Here's how the LiverUp! Cleanse works. Just follow these five steps:

1. Start each day by drinking 2 glasses of water with the juice of half a lime or lemon (not bottled lemon juice) to support your cleansing efforts. Excellent liver detoxifiers, lemons contain lots of vitamin C, which helps your body make glutathione—and that helps your liver detoxify harmful chemicals. Then, if you can, wait 30 to 45 minutes before eating breakfast. During the day, you'll continue to drink lots of water to help support your liver's detox process. Plus, every day you'll have a cup of dandelion root tea and take a milk thistle supplement.

2. Over the course of each day, choose at least one food from each category of "The Cleanse at a Glance" (see page 90). You can use the recipes in Chapter 9 and follow the menu plans in the Appendix, or you can get creative and devise your own dishes, using the foods on the chart. You can make any combinations you prefer. The key is to
(continued on page 92)

{The Cleanse at a Glance

FOOD GROUP	SERVING SIZE	EXAMPLES
Water	Eight to ten 8-ounce glasses	Water with lemon, lime, or a few berries
Cruciferous Vegetables	$\frac{1}{2}$ cup cooked or 1 cup raw	Broccoli, broccolini, broccoli rabe, cauliflower, kohlrabi, turnips, rutabaga, parsnips, daikon
Dark Leafy Greens	$\frac{1}{2}$ cup cooked or 1 cup raw	Kale, chard, watercress, bok choy, arugula, cabbage, Chinese cabbage, collard greens, spinach, Brussels sprouts, cilantro, beet greens, radish greens, escarole, dandelion greens, endive
Sea Vegetables	2–4 tablespoons	Kelp, dulse flakes, wakame, arame
Sprouted Seeds, Nuts, Beans, and Grains	1 cup	Broccoli seeds, lentil, mung beans, chickpeas, barley
Sulfur-Rich Foods	$\frac{1}{4}$ cup onions, shallots, or leeks; 1–2 cloves garlic; 1–2 eggs; 1–2 artichoke hearts; $\frac{1}{2}$ cup mushrooms	Onions, garlic, eggs, artichokes, medicinal mushrooms
Fruits	1 apple or $\frac{1}{2}$ cup berries	Berries, apples, lemons, limes
Prebiotic-Rich Foods	$\frac{1}{2}$ cup cooked or 1 cup raw	Asparagus, burdock root, chicory, dandelion root, beets, Jerusalem artichoke, leeks, cruciferous vegetables (see list above)
Cultured Foods	$\frac{1}{2}$ cup sauerkraut and kimchi; 1–2 tablespoons miso	Raw sauerkraut, kimchi, miso

Seeds, Nuts, and Nut Butters	1–2 ounces	Walnuts, almonds, pumpkin seeds, sesame seeds, sunflower seeds, almond butter, cashew butter
Healthy Fats	2 tablespoons seeds; 1/2 avocado; 1–2 tablespoons oil	Flax seeds; chia seeds; hemp seeds; coconut oil; avocado; cold-pressed, unrefined, extra virgin olive oil
Herbs	Aim for 2 herbs per day	Ginger, cumin, coriander, cilantro, cardamom, cinnamon, fennel, cayenne, turmeric, parsley
Protein	4 ounces animal protein; 1 scoop whey or hemp protein powder; 1–2 teaspoons microalgae; 2 tablespoons hemp seeds	Wild-caught fish, grass-fed beef, free-range chicken, turkey, lamb, whey protein powder, microalgae, hemp powder, hemp seeds
Sweet Potatoes	1/2 large; 1 small	An occasional treat

Foods to Maximize. Choose one serving from each of the groups. You don't have to *eat* all your veggies—you can *drink* them, too! In Chapter 9, you'll find recipes for easy fruit-and-veggie smoothies that count toward your daily selections. Also, one serving of food in more than one group can count for both groups.

Foods to Avoid or Minimize. Try to stay away from these groups of food. Later in the chapter, you'll learn all about how they can sabotage your health.

- Processed foods, refined carbs, and sugar
- Wheat and all gluten-containing grains
- Dairy
- Trans fats
- Caffeine and alcohol
- Soy products
- All sweeteners except stevia (very small amounts of honey, maple syrup, or agave nectar are allowed during the optional fast)

incorporate one or more foods from each section over the course of your three meals for the day.

3. Slow down. Make these 12 days a time to reconnect with your body and heal your mind. Try some of the many suggestions you'll find in Chapter 7.

4. Move. Yoga is an especially healing practice during your cleanse. Even if you're a novice, you'll find the illustrated routine in Chapter 8 easy to follow. Try to commit to 30 minutes a day on the mat.

5. Write. Use the journal on pages 312 and 313 or your own notebook or smartphone to record your food choices, your yoga and meditation practices, and your thoughts and reflections as you journey through these 12 days.

Healing Foods— Detox Powerhouses

The foods that make up the LiverUp! Cleanse are nutritious and healing. Let's take a look at the science behind these foods to see why they'll help make these 12 days transformative. First we'll talk a bit about water.

Water

Water is the largest single component of which humans are built—it makes up 55 to 60 percent of your body and 70 to 80 percent of your brain. After oxygen, your body needs water more than any other substance, including food, just to survive. On average, we lose approximately 2½ quarts of water a day just by breathing, sweating, urinating, and defecating.

Most of us don't drink enough water, and even mild dehydration can cause us to experience sluggish thinking, poor digestion, slowed metabolism, and fatigue. Lack of water is the primary trigger of daytime fatigue.[1] Because water flushes toxins and waste products from your body, you feel more energized and alert when your body is fully hydrated. Since water is crucial for every bodily operation, when you become dehydrated, your body senses trouble and instinctively begins to ration it to each organ, seeking to store fluids between tissues and cells, which causes fluid retention and excess water weight. And when you're chronically dehydrated, you store excess fat. Water helps with detoxing—through your kidneys, colon, liver, and skin.

So how much water is enough? Usually eight to ten 8-ounce glasses will do the trick. When you're cleansing, however, drink half your body weight in ounces. For example, if you weigh 160 pounds, you will want to drink 80 ounces of water, or ten 8-ounce glasses.

When you exercise or the weather is hot and dry, increase your water intake. When you sweat and lose fluids, energy levels can drop. Hydration helps keep your body in homeostasis, allowing it to maintain a steady metabolism, efficient transportation of nutrients to your cells, and even steady levels of blood sugar.

The key is to drink the appropriate amount of water for your body type, your weight, and your exercise level. Remember, too much water can cause problems, too. You'll be surprised at how much more energy, less joint and muscular pain, less hunger, and perhaps even less anxiety

Downing Your Daily Quota

What's the best way to drink your water? Here are a few tips.

• Drink room temperature water in between meals—drinking ice water with meals dilutes important digestive enzymes. Ice water needs to be warmed by your body, which takes energy and hampers your digestion.
• Drink a cup of hot water with lemon after a meal to support digestion.
• Consume more water-based foods—cabbage, lettuces, citrus, and broth-based soups.
• For a bit of flavor and added nutrients, add a splash of lemon or pure cranberry juice, some thin cucumber slices, or a few frozen berries to your water.

you may experience when you drink the right amount of water. It's all about hydrating properly so your liver, kidneys, lymph, and colon can do their jobs and detox your body.

Crucifers

In the world of vegetables, these are the superstars. They support your liver in filtering every single bite you eat, aiding detoxification by helping your liver convert fat-soluble toxins into water-soluble substances that can be excreted via your kidneys.

Crucifers contain vital phytonutrients—flavonoids, carotenoids, sulforaphane, and indoles—to help your liver neutralize chemicals, pesticides, drugs, and carcinogens; to disarm free radicals; and to prevent cellular degeneration. That protects your body against cancer and other age-related diseases. Here's how.

Flavonoids, naturally occurring plant pigments that help reduce

{Go Organic!

According to the Environmental Working Group, these fruits and veggies make up the Dirty Dozen Plus. Nonorganic produce contains the highest amounts of pesticides and other toxins, and this list calls out the worst offenders, so try to buy organic whenever you can, especially for the following.

1. Apples
2. Celery
3. Cherry tomatoes
4. Cucumbers
5. Grapes
6. Hot peppers
7. Nectarines (imported)
8. Peaches
9. Potatoes
10. Spinach
11. Strawberries
12. Sweet bell peppers

+PLUS

- Collards and kale
- Summer squash and zucchini

your risk of cancer, heart disease, asthma, and stroke, may play a role in protecting your brain. Like other antioxidants, they neutralize cell-damaging free radicals. But they don't stop there. Scientists have found that certain flavonoids have antihistamine, antimicrobial, and memory- and mood-enhancing properties.[2]

Sulforaphane is a sulfur-based chemical that stimulates Phase Two enzymes, which are essential in neutralizing free radicals and carcinogens, thus reducing the cellular oxidation that contributes to cancer. In boosting these enzymes, sulforaphane plays a critical role in preventing the disease. If cancer is present, sulforaphane, with the help of other antioxidants, causes cancer cells to self-destruct in a process called apoptosis. Plus, sulforaphane helps prevent cancerous changes in cells by boosting your immune system. It increases the killer immune cells and stimulates other parts of your immune system.[3]

Carotenoids are yellow, orange, red, and green pigments in plants like carrots, sweet potatoes, winter squash, kale, watermelon, apricots, and tomatoes. Your body uses some of these pigments to make vitamin A. Carotenoids are potent fat-soluble antioxidants that help prevent free radical damage to your cells and support your immune system.

Indoles are sulfur-containing phytonutrients that modulate the activity of enzymes in your liver, enhancing natural detoxification pathways. These protective phytochemicals help your liver by inhibiting carcinogen-activating Phase One liver enzymes while inducing the carcinogen-detoxifying Phase Two enzymes. As we've learned, Phase Two enzymes convert dangerous compounds, such as toxins, hormones, and xenoestrogens, into less-toxic compounds that can safely be eliminated by your body.[4]

In addition to their detoxification qualities, cruciferous vegetables contain high levels of nutrients, including vitamins C, A, and K, as well as calcium, magnesium, potassium, phosphorous, sulfur, and fiber. These assist your liver in both Phase One and Phase Two detoxification.

And when it comes to cruciferous vegetables, daikon gets the gold star, providing some of the best food-based digestive enzymes available.

The root and leaves contain the enzymes diastase, amylase, and esterase, which help you digest fats, carbohydrates, and proteins all at once. In addition, daikon's sulfur compounds help increase the flow of bile, further assisting your liver in breaking down and absorbing fats and supporting digestion. Daikon is a great natural decongestant, with enzymes that help open up your respiratory system and dissolve mucus. Plus, it contains antimicrobial, antiviral, anti-inflammatory, and sulfur-based compounds, and its antioxidants may help to fight damage caused by free radicals. You can try juicing it, too. Its phenolic compounds help prevent the formation of carcinogens in your stomach in response to foods made with hydrogenated oils (found in many processed sweets and chips) and sodium nitrite (found in hot dogs and cured meats). Finally, daikon acts as a healthy, potassium-preserving diuretic, activating your kidneys and allowing them to release excess fluid. It promotes complete urination and reduces swelling from edema.

Dark Leafy Greens

Raw, baked, sautéed, or steamed, dark green leafy vegetables provide more nutrients, calorie for calorie, than any other land-based food. These members of the brassica or cabbage family are loaded with minerals and vitamins. They provide the same powerful anticancer compounds, such as phytochemcials, that function as antioxidants to help protect and cleanse your body of harmful substances.[5]

Dark leafy greens contain high levels of sulfur, which supports your liver in its detoxification process, triggering it to remove free radicals and other toxic chemicals. These greens are also high in fiber, which helps cleanse your intestinal tract and flush toxins from your body.

Plus, green leafy vegetables are high in calcium, as well as vitamins A, C, and K. Vitamin K activates a compound called osteocalcin, which anchors calcium molecules, enabling calcium and many minerals to find their way into your bones. These amazing plants sprout shoots that take nutrients from the soil, along with the sun's life-giving energy, and transform them into large, flat leaves. Through photosynthesis, these leaves take in carbon dioxide and release oxygen into the air. When we consume these large leaves, we're also consuming rich chlorophyll and oxygen-promoting nutrients. No wonder we feel energized after a plateful of these power-packed greens. And while they're all superstars, a few should be mentioned, because they're often overlooked.

Kale, Brussels Sprouts, and Cabbage. These are among my most prized greens—though kale gets most of its attention by adorning meat and vegetable platters and Brussels sprouts are shunned for their smell. Along with other brassica vegetables, they contain powerful antioxidants and phytochemicals, along with sulforaphane. All three vegetables provide significant levels of vitamins A (as beta-carotene), C, and K. Kale, in particular, is loaded with calcium and iron.

Dandelion. Another superstar, dandelion has been used worldwide for detoxification for centuries. The scientific name for dandelion is *Taraxacum officinale*, which means "official remedy for the disorders."

While we may consider dandelion a weed, it is, in fact, a powerful herb. In *The Natural Physician's Healing Therapies*, Mark Stengler, ND, writes that dandelion ranks as high as milk thistle as the most effective and recommended herb to support liver detoxification. One of dandelion's chemical components, taraxacin, is believed to stimulate the digestive organs and trigger the liver and gallbladder to release bile, which supports digestion and fat absorption.[6]

Sea Vegetables

Sea vegetables, among the oldest inhabitants of the earth, contain many of the essential nutrients your body needs, including vitamins, amino acids, calcium, iodine, and iron. They also contain the broadest range of minerals of any organism.[7] After all, seaweeds are soaked in mineral-rich seawater. They detoxify your body by preventing assimilation of heavy metals, such as cadmium, as well as other environmental toxins. Studies at McGill University have revealed that a compound in brown algae (arame, kombu, and wakame) reduced the uptake of radioactive particles into bone.[8] Plus, seaweeds are being used in the treatment of cancer and fibroid tumors. According to ancient Chinese texts, all swelling can be relieved by seaweed.[9]

Sprouted Seeds, Nuts, Beans, and Grains

The energy contained in a seed, grain, nut, or legume is ignited through soaking and sprouting. And those sprouts are superhigh in enzymes, proteins that act as catalysts for all of your body's functions. Some experts estimate that sprouts may contain 100 times more enzymes than uncooked fruits and vegetables.[10]

The sprouting process actually enhances the nutritional value of the existing protein present in seeds, nuts, beans, and grains. The amino acid lysine, which supports a healthy immune system and helps prevent cold sores, is a good example.[11] Sprouting also increases the fiber content substantially. And fiber helps to flush out fat that your body breaks down before it can be reabsorbed through the walls of your intestines, binding to fats and toxins and escorting them out through your colon.[12]

Sprouting also increases the vitamin content of vitamins A, B complex, C, and E. Research shows that during the sprouting process mung bean sprouts may increase in vitamin B_1, vitamin B_2, and niacin by more than 200 percent.[13] Broccoli sprouts may help protect your stomach from gastritis, ulcers, and cancer. Researchers at Johns Hopkins University have shown that small quantities of fresh broccoli sprouts contain as much cancer protection as larger amounts of the mature vegetable. Less than 2 ounces of sprouts contains significant concentrations of sulforaphane, which triggers your body's natural cancer protection resources. Scientists also found that broccoli sprouts appear to be an exceptionally rich source of compounds that enhance the activity of your liver's Phase Two enzymes that help detox your body of chemicals and carcinogens.[14]

Importantly, sprouts are alkalizing to your body. The sprouting process stimulates minerals to bind with the protein in seeds, grains, nuts, and beans, making both minerals and proteins more usable. Alkaline minerals, such as calcium and magnesium, help to balance your body chemistry. Many illnesses, including cancer, have been linked to excess acidity in the body.[15]

Sprout Your Own Sprouts!

Sprouts are a simple, nutritious way to grow your own food in any season or environment. And when you grow your own, you'll be consuming pesticide-, additive-, and chemical-free whole foods that help detox your body. Best of all, they're really easy to grow.

1. Place 1 to 2 tablespoons of seeds in a glass canning jar and cover the opening with cheesecloth or another porous material. Secure the cloth with a rubber band. Fill the jar with filtered water and let the seeds soak overnight.

2. In the morning, drain off the water. The cloth or porous plastic top will keep the seeds in the jar. Rinse the seeds with water again, and drain them.

3. Put the container on its side, out of direct sunlight, in a spot with a temperature of about 70°F. Rinse and drain the seeds twice daily.

4. Continue this cycle until all of your sprouts have been harvested. Depending on what seeds, beans, or grains you use, your sprouts will be ready to harvest in 2 to 5 days. When they're 1 or 2 inches long, put them in the light to green them up.

You can rinse out the hulls or put some water in the jar, remove the cheesecloth, and skim them off the top of the water with a spoon. The hulls aren't harmful to eat, but removing them minimizes spoilage when you store your sprouts. Once harvested, store your sprouts in an airtight container in your refrigerator. They'll keep for 1 to 2 weeks.

You can order broccoli seeds online at vitacost.com and find mung beans, lentils, aduki beans, chickpeas, and grains at any health food store.

Sulfur-Rich Foods

Sulfur supports the liver's Phase Two Detoxification process, helping to convert oxidized chemicals into nontoxic compounds. The LiverUp! Cleanse includes many delicious, sulfur-rich foods.

Garlic. Garlic is one of the oldest land-based medicinal foods on the planet, with benefits that have been documented in more than 1,000 studies. It contains an active sulfur-based compound called allicin, which is critical in supporting your liver's detoxification process. It helps your liver rid your body of mercury, certain food additives, and the hormone estrogen. Plus, it works as a mild antimicrobial agent.

Allicin also helps defend your body against heart disease, cancer, and other chronic diseases by helping to clean plaque and cholesterol buildup from your arteries and by providing both anticancer and antioxidant properties that help detoxify your body of harmful substances. In a large study published in the *Journal of the Royal College of Physicians,* garlic supplements lowered participants' total cholesterol by 12 percent after only 4 weeks of treatment. Plus, garlic lowered LDL (bad) cholesterol by 4 to 15 percent without lowering HDL (good) cholesterol. In many cases, garlic actually raised HDL by as much as 20 percent, while lowering triglycerides.[16]

Onions, shallots, and leeks. Like garlic, onions and their relatives contain a treasure chest of smelly sulfur compounds that support your liver in its production of glutathione, the compound in every cell of your body that neutralizes free radicals, keeps your cells running smoothly, lowers both blood lipids (fat) and blood pressure, and supports your liver in removing toxic chemicals. Like garlic, onions are antioxidant, antibiotic, antiviral, and anti-inflammatory. They contain quercetin, an anti-inflammatory compound used to treat cancer, heart disease, and many allergies.

Eggs. Eggs provide some of the highest-quality protein, containing all eight essential amino acids, cholesterol, and the essential nutrient choline. Your liver needs these essential amino acids to perform its Phase Two detoxification process, and it needs cholesterol to make bile. Choline, a coenzyme needed for metabolism, exists in all living cells but is probably best known as a major part of lecithin—the emulsifier that keeps fats and cholesterol from clumping together in your blood. It's found in the egg yolk and is important to both your liver and your entire body. It helps heal and support your liver, protecting it from a wide range of toxic substances, while detoxifying heavy metals.

If you eat animal protein, free-range eggs from hens that truly roam freely are an ideal food. Eggs provide some of best—and least expensive—protein available. These eggs are often found at your local farmers' market or through your local CSA (community-supported agriculture). If you eat eggs, take the time to locate a farmer who raises chickens that are truly free roaming and free to eat pesticide- and chemical-free plants, bugs, and worms.

Artichokes. Artichokes are particularly high in antioxidants, in the form of vitamin C, and phytonutrients, which protect cells against the attack of free radicals. Two of these phytonutrients, cynarin and silymarin, have been shown to nourish your liver, increase bile production, and prevent gallstones. An Indian study suggests that silymarin, the active ingredient in milk thistle, may also help control blood sugar in type 2 diabetics.[17]

These phytonutrients have been shown to lower cholesterol and triglycerides in your bloodstream and to increase the relative level of high-density lipoprotein (HDL), or "good" cholesterol.[18] Your liver uses cholesterol to make bile acids, then stores them in your gallbladder. By increasing the production of bile acids, artichokes help reduce LDL (bad) cholesterol in your bloodstream. And bile also helps your body efficiently digest fats and absorb fat-soluble vitamins. This may be why ancient cultures used artichokes so often as a remedy for indigestion.

Medicinal Mushrooms. Maitake, shiitake, and reishi mushrooms are thought to provide significant healing nutrients that nourish and support your immune system. As they live off trees and decaying organic matter, they absorb and release toxins. Just as green leafy plants release oxygen, these fungi may work at absorbing and eliminating toxins in your body. Researchers at the University of California, Davis, Medical School found that these mushrooms possess compounds that provide antitumor, cholesterol-lowering, and virus-inhibiting effects.[19] They help boost your body's immune system and help prevent heart disease by lowering cholesterol levels.

Perhaps most importantly, these mushrooms contain a powerful antioxidant called L-ergothioneine, which neutralizes free radicals while increasing enzymes that boost antioxidant activity. Researchers at the Touro College of Pharmacy in New York City found that L-ergothioneine supports the body in maintaining adequate levels of vitamin E, vitamin C, and glutathione. This appears to increase respiration and the oxidation of fat, which can contribute to increased energy and exercise capacity. Plus, these fungi protect the mitochondria in your cells from environmental ultraviolet radiation damage.[20]

Fruits

One or two servings of fruit a day can be an important part of your healthy cleanse. Apples and berries, in particular, are higher in antioxidants and lower in sugars than other fruits.

Berries. Blueberries, strawberries, raspberries, and cranberries are among nature's superfoods because they contain phytochemicals—antioxidant-rich plant compounds that help your liver protect your body from free radicals and oxidative stress, which have been linked to chronic diseases and aging.[21] In a number of studies, berries have been shown to support the cardiovascular system, improve brain function, and slow the proliferation of cancer cells.

Berries contain the anti-inflammatory plant compounds and beneficial antioxidants anthocyanin and polyphenol. Remember that inflammation and oxidative stress are involved in atherosclerotic heart disease, when plaque forms on the inside of your artery walls. Inflammation and oxidative stress are also factors in cancer, diabetes, Parkinson's, Alzheimer's, and arthritis.[22]

Recent research supports these findings. In 2013, researchers at the Harvard School of Public Health reported that eating anthocyanin-rich strawberries or blueberries—as few as three $\frac{1}{2}$-cup servings per week—appeared to reduce the risk of heart attack in women by as much as 33 percent, by regulating fatty acid metabolism and fats in the bloodstream and by preventing the deposition of plaque in the arteries.[23]

In addition, the anthocyanin and polyphenols found in berries have been shown to inhibit the proliferation of cancer cells in the liver.[24] These compounds have also been shown to inhibit the growth of tumors caused by certain carcinogens, causing cancer cell death (apoptosis) in the lab—with no change to healthy, normal cells.[25]

Apples. Like berries, apples contain phytochemicals that reduce oxidative stress—the damage done to cells and DNA by oxidation, which has been linked to many diseases. Like berries, apples possess many of these powerful antioxidants—they're topped only by cranberries for their antioxidant capacity.

Also like berries, apples contain powerful phenolic compounds, including flavonoids, that fight cancer and other inflammatory diseases. They also contain pectin, a valuable source of soluble fiber that can lower LDL (bad) cholesterol, help regulate blood sugar, help eliminate toxic buildup, and help to cleanse your intestines.

Prebiotic-Rich Foods

Prebiotics are indigestible fibers that feed your beneficial gut flora, known as probiotics. Probiotics are living microorganisms that support your health and wellbeing. Prebiotics are nonliving dietary fibers that help probiotics grow and flourish. Prebiotics can't be digested or absorbed in your intestinal tract, but the microflora in your large intestines and colon thrive on them. Two of the most significant prebiotics are inulin and oligofructose.

Prebiotics are found in asparagus, leeks, cruciferous vegetables, and several root vegetables—burdock, chicory, dandelion, beets, and Jerusalem artichoke. Let's take a look at a few of the lesser known roots—burdock, chicory, and Jerusalem artichoke.

Burdock is a very long, skinny root that can grow up to 2 feet long. Because of its length, many Eastern practitioners believe it to be grounding for the body and mind. Sold in most health food stores, it is delicious in a stir-fry or stew. Just make sure to scrub all the dirt off.

Chicory root was used by both ancient Romans and Egyptians to cleanse the liver and blood, as it increases production of bile. Today, its notoriety comes from the fact that the root contains the highest concentration of inulin.

Jerusalem artichokes, often called sunchokes, are neither from Jerusalem nor are artichokes. Rather they are tubers in the sunflower family and contain substantial amounts of inulin. When they are roasted or sautéed, they have a slightly sweet, crisp, nutty flavor and are delicious in soups or as a substitute for potatoes.

Cultured Foods

These include kimchi—a traditional Korean dish made of fermented cabbage, radish, garlic, red pepper, onion, seafood, ginger, and salt—and sauerkraut. Kimchi is a great winter food—it helps keep the body warm—and sauerkraut is a similar dish that is believed to have originated in China. Legend has it that laborers building the Great Wall of China over 2,000 years ago preserved their cabbage with rice wine so they'd be able to eat it beyond its growing season. One thousand years later, it was brought to eastern Europe as sauerkraut, which is German for "sour cabbage."

The healing properties of kimchi and sauerkraut begin with cabbage—one of the healthiest foods. Cabbage and other cruciferous vegetables provide powerful phytochemicals and flavonoids that support your liver's Phase Two detox process by increasing the production of enzymes that neutralize free radicals and help fight carcinogens. The flavonoids in cabbage provide additional antioxidants that lower LDL (bad) cholesterol while supporting your liver against toxins.

The powerful nutrition of both kimchi and sauerkraut is multiplied by fermentation, an ancient form of preservation in which food is naturally transformed by microorganisms that break down all the food's carbohydrates and protein. Miso is another example. It's made of fermented soybeans along with brown rice, white rice, barley, or buckwheat.

Almost all fermented foods promote health and healing because of both the fermentation process and the quality of the foods from which they're made. And they may help with digestion. Healthy bacteria, such as lactobacilli, are essential to the fermentation process, and kimchi and miso, in particular, provide a plethora of these probiotics. Remember that probiotics play a pivotal role in supporting your body's immune system at the cellular level, increasing antibodies when you have infections and helping to reduce inflammation. Probiotics are key in maintaining a healthy digestive system, which in turn supports your immune and detoxification systems.

Healthy Fats

Healthy fats are essential for a healthy liver—and for your well-being in general. The ratio of omega-6 fatty acids to omega-3 fatty acids in your diet is critical to your health. Much of the standard American diet is comprised of excessive amounts of omega-6 compared to omega-3 fatty acids. This extreme imbalance contributes to the development of inflammation-triggered diseases. Here are your best choices for healthy fats.

Flax seeds. Flax seeds are a great source of omega-3 essential fatty acids, which help lower triglycerides, reduce plaque formation, support brain function, and regulate hormone levels. They support cell membranes, making them more pliant so that neurotransmitters, our communication chemicals, can enter and exit our cells more fluidly. Neurotransmitters such as serotonin and dopamine affect your mood and sense of well-being, so when these chemicals flow more easily, we feel better emotionally.

According to Bernadine Healy, MD, former director of the National Institutes of Health (NIH), and Joseph R. Hibbeln, MD, acting chief of the National Institute on Alcohol Abuse and Alcoholism at the NIH, consuming these fats in proper proportion may actually relieve many health conditions.[26] Adding foods high in omega-3 fatty acids, such as flax seeds, they say, supports your liver in helping your body reduce inflammation, which protects you from a host of inflammation-generated disease. In addition, flax seeds provide both soluble and insoluble fiber, as well as lignans, estrogen-regulating substances with antiviral, antibacterial, and antifungal properties.

Hemp Seeds. Hemp seeds contain both omega-6 and omega-3 fatty acids, supporting cardiovascular health.

Research confirms that "clean" omega-6 fats—those that are not heated, refined, or processed—lower LDL (bad) cholesterol. And the omega-3s in hemp lower triglycerides, blood cholesterol levels, plaque accumulation, and inflammation. They contain about 25 percent protein, between 10 and 15 percent fiber, and a host of minerals.

Chia Seeds. Chia seeds, cultivated for thousands of years and a staple of the Central American Aztec and Mayan diets, were recognized not only for their nutritional qualities, but also for their energizing properties. Much like quinoa, the propagation of chia seeds was threatened with the arrival of Spanish conquistadors. The invading Europeans barred any foods linked to traditional Aztecan culture. Fortunately, a few tribes defied that order, so we have the seeds today.

Like flax, chia seeds are a beneficial source of omega-3s. However, chia seeds contain much higher amounts of antioxidants than flax seeds do, so they can be stored for a long time without becoming rancid. Plus, chia seeds are high in protein and fiber—3 tablespoons contain 5 grams of protein, 200 milligrams of calcium, 10 grams of healthy fat, and 12 grams of fiber.

Coconut Oil. Though North Americans have been phobic about saturated fats since the 1980s, coconut oil is an extremely healthy saturated fat. Your body needs quality fats for a host of processes, and saturated fats, in the form of medium-chain triglycerides (MCTs), are hugely beneficial.

One unique property of the MCTs in coconut oil is that they require less energy and fewer enzymes for digestion than other fats, because their molecules are smaller. MCTs are broken down almost immediately by enzymes in your saliva and gastric juices, so pancreatic fat-digesting enzymes are not essential, as they are for the digestion of longer-chain fats. This results in less strain on your pancreas and digestive system, allowing your liver to do its job more efficiently and effectively.[27]

Other types of dietary fats must be broken down in your intestines and made into a different type of fat in order to be transported in your blood so they can be used for energy. MCTs are broken down to medium-chain fatty acids and absorbed from your intestinal walls and transported directly to your liver. There they are converted into energy for the entire body. And because they're easily absorbed by the energy-producing structures of your cells, your metabolism increases. This burst of energy has a stimulating effect on your entire body. Coconut oil also improves digestive functioning, so your system more easily absorbs amino acids, vitamins, and minerals.

In *Eat Fat, Lose Fat,* author Mary Enig explains that the predominant medium-chain fatty acid in coconut oil is lauric acid, which possesses the same antibacterial, antiviral, antifungal, antiparasitic, and anti-inflammatory properties as mother's milk, protecting your body from harmful microorganisms.[28] It's important to consume virgin or extra-virgin coconut oil, which has all of its healing properties intact.

Avocado. Avocado contains a monounsaturated fat that's rich in oleic acid, an omega-9 fat also found in olive and macadamia nut oils. Oleic acid has been shown to lower LDL (bad) cholesterol and raise HDL (good) cholesterol. In addition to monounsaturated fat, avocados have a small amount of saturated fat, which has been shown to protect against atherosclerosis, keeping arteries supple and free of artery-blocking toxicity. In a UCLA study of 11 healthy men between the ages of 18 and 35, eating half an avocado with a burger, rather than a burger alone, curbed the production of compounds that contribute to inflammation, a risk factor associated with heart disease.[29]

Avocados contain glutathione, an essential nutrient for liver health. It blocks many carcinogens and helps your liver detoxify synthetic chemicals. Plus, avocados are a great source of fiber, which makes them a beautiful cleansing food.

Cold-Pressed, Unrefined Extra-Virgin Olive Oil. When olive oil is cold pressed and unrefined, all its vitamins, essential fatty acids, antioxidants, and other nutrients are preserved. With the best oils, the olives are picked by hand and the oil is separated without heat, hot water, or solvents, and it's left unfiltered. The first pressing produces the highest quality oil, called "extra virgin."

Cold-pressed, unrefined, extra-virgin olive oil is high in phenols, the same antioxidant, anti-inflammatory, cancer-fighting plant compounds found in berries and apples. Phenols, which are water soluble, are washed away during processing—that's why unrefined oil is so beneficial. It's also high in oleic acid, the same monounsaturated fat found in avocados that has been associated with cardiovascular health. Oleic acid has been shown to lower LDL (bad) cholesterol while increasing HDL (good) cholesterol.

In a study of almost 200 healthy men from six countries, participants consumed either virgin olive oil (high in polyphenols), refined olive oil (low in polyphenols), or a mixture of the two oils in equal parts. Groups consumed 25 milliliters of one of these daily for 3 weeks, followed by the other olive oils in a randomly assigned sequence. Olive oils with greater polyphenol content increased HDL (good) cholesterol levels and decreased markers of oxidation. The *Annals of Internal Medicine* cites a study showing that a daily dose of phenol-rich oil reduced cardio-vascular risk factors and improved levels of the antioxidant glutathione. Moreover, daily consumption of olive oil supported the liver in decreasing oxidative stress in the body, raising HDL cholesterol levels and reducing the oxidative damage to lipids.[30]

Herbs

Variety is the spice of life, and herbs add that variety to everyday foods. But they can also be medicinal, especially to your liver. Here's a look at some of the most beneficial herbs.

Ginger. Ginger is known as the "universal remedy" in Ayurveda, India's ancient "science of life." It's full of antioxidants called gingerols, which possess anti-inflammatory, antiviral, and antimicrobial properties. Ginger supports detoxification by nourishing your liver, promoting circulation, unclogging blocked arteries, and lowering blood cholesterol by as much as 30 percent.[31]

Ginger aids in digestion by supplying compounds that mimic your digestive enzymes, helping you to metabolize protein-rich foods with less effort from your liver and digestive system. It's been used for centuries to treat upset stomach and nausea. Fresh ginger can be used in any recipe to add a bit of zip and spice. Blend some into your smoothies, grate some over sweet potatoes, or steep thin slices in hot water for a warming tea.

Cumin. Cumin is a seed of a small flowering herb in the parsley family. This traditional herbal remedy has many uses. In Ayurveda, it's a healing herb used for digestive disorders—flatulence, indigestion, diarrhea, nausea, morning sickness, and dyspepsia. The seeds are boiled in water to make a tea—1 teaspoon of seeds to 1 cup water.

In one Indian study, cumin was shown to boost the liver's detoxification power while stimulating the secretion of enzymes from the pancreas, which helps your system absorb nutrients.[32] Another Indian study has revealed that cumin seeds are more powerful antioxidants than vitamin C, scavenging free radicals and reducing total cholesterol, triglycerides, and pancreatic inflammatory markers in diabetic rats.[33]

⌄ **Coriander (Cilantro Leaves).** Coriander is both an herb and a spice. Its parsleylike leaves are considered an herb, and this form is often called cilantro. The seeds, which look like light brown peppercorns, are a fragrant spice and taste like a mixture of sweet orange peel and sage. Both the seeds and the leaves are considered powerful detox foods, as they promote healthy liver function. Coriander is rich in many important vitamins, including folic acid, vitamin A, beta-carotene, and vitamin C, all of which are essential for optimum health.

Coriander seeds have been shown to help the liver lower blood lipids among those with obesity and diabetes, lowering triglycerides and LDL (bad) cholesterol, while increasing HDL (good) cholesterol.[34] Fresh cilantro leaves have been shown to help remove heavy metals from the body. According to research presented at the University of Geneva, cilantro can mobilize mercury, cadmium, lead, and aluminum that's been stored in the brain, spinal cord, and central nervous system and flush them out through your body's elimination systems.[35]

⌄ **Cardamom.** A member of the ginger family, cardamom improves digestion by stimulating the flow of bile, which is critical in fat metabolism. It accelerates the gastric emptying rate, relaxing the stomach valves that prevent food from entering the small intestine, allowing nutrients to pass on to the small intestine without excess effort.

Cardamom is also a powerful mucus destroyer. As with all aromatics, cardamom opens your pores, helps reduce low-grade fevers, and cleanses your lymphatic system.

⌄ **Cayenne.** Cayenne, a powerful anti-inflammatory and natural detoxer that stimulates your circulatory system, increases the pulse of your lymphatic and digestive rhythms, thus heating your body. Its hotness comes from a high concentration of capsicum, a substance that has been used to stimulate circulation for centuries. The capsicum in cayenne helps your blood flow efficiently, stimulates your body's metabolic rate, and helps clean fat from your arteries. A natural energizer, cayenne stimulates your digestive tract, increasing the flow of enzyme production and gastric juices, enhancing your body's ability to metabolize food and toxins. Cayenne is also helpful for relieving flatulence. It stimulates intestinal peristaltic motion, aiding in both assimilation and elimination. And like cardamom, cayenne aids in breaking up and moving congested mucus, easing cold and flu symptoms.

Cinnamon. Cinnamon has been used for centuries for flavor and medicine. Its healing properties include its ability to (1) keep sticky platelets from forming clots in your arteries, (2) boost metabolism, and (3) prevent candida, the microorganism that causes yeast overgrowth in your body. In addition, it appears that cinnamon may help lower blood sugar.

Some cinnamon undergoes radiation during processing, which can reduce its vitamin and antioxidant content, as well as promote free radicals that are potentially harmful. Consider purchasing organic cinnamon.

Fennel. Like cardamom and cayenne, fennel contains essential oils that help support your digestive process. They do this by prompting the secretion of gastric juices, lowering inflammation in your digestive tract, diminishing acid production, and helping your body absorb nutrients more efficiently.

Turmeric. Another member of the ginger family, turmeric may be the ultimate spice powerhouse. A staple in Indian cooking, turmeric gives food a distinctive flavor and is an important spice in curry.

While it's made up of many compounds, turmeric's bright yellow color comes from curcuminoids, one of the most important of which is curcumin. Curcumin is a powerful antioxidant and anti-inflammatory, shown to be healing for your liver. It aids in your liver's detoxification process, thus purifying and strengthening your whole body.[36]

Protein

After water, protein is the most abundant substance in your body. It's made from amino acids—protein's building blocks. Your body can produce just over half of the 20 amino acids it uses for building new cells, maintaining tissues, and synthesizing new proteins it needs to perform basic functions. The other nine amino acids must come from food, so they're considered to be essential.

Unlike carbohydrates and fats, your body can't store protein, so you need to supply your body's protein needs daily—and if you eat more than your body can handle, you must dispose of that excess daily, as well.

The most convenient source for complete protein is animal foods. But the meat that we eat today is vastly different than the meat humans have been eating for 99 percent of our life span on the planet. And we're eating significantly larger portions than we ever have. Because your body can only assimilate what it needs, it must work hard at breaking down the excess and eliminating it. This can cause calcium loss, increase your need for fluids, and make your kidneys work harder.

That's why some people choose vegetable sources for their daily protein, so the LiverUp! Cleanse offers options for omnivores and herbivores. The key is to listen to your body. Experiment to see what protein sources make you feel energized, satisfied, and balanced.

Animal Protein

For more than 2 million years, our ancestors ate a diet that consisted largely of what they could hunt (wild game) and what they could gather (roots, berries, nuts, wild vegetables, and tart fruit when it was available). For most of our evolution, we've been eating hormone-, antibiotic-, and pesticide-free, naturally organic, and entirely range-fed animal protein. Over that same time period, our diet was rich in fat: saturated fat, monounsaturated fat, omega-3 fats, balanced omega-6 fats, and a variety of fat-soluble nutrients. During that time, the human brain has enlarged and developed rapidly.

In *Primal Body, Primal Mind,* author and nutritional therapist Nora Gedgaudas writes that humans would never have survived without animal protein and its valuable dietary fat.[37] For most of our existence, we've depended on nutrient-rich dietary fats in the form of meats, fatty fish, and bone marrow for at least 60 percent of our caloric consumption—without detriment to our hearts. It wasn't until 1912 that heart disease was even recorded, but by the 1950s, just 40 years later, it was one of the leading causes of death among Americans. What happened during those 40 years? The emergence of the factory farm and industrialized food: processed foods; hydrogenated oils; sugar; refined carbohydrates; high-fructose corn syrup; and factory-raised grain- or corn-fed cows, chickens, and fish. Much of our diet today is composed of this low-quality, industrialized food. And our health is declining as a result.

Given our history, many health practitioners believe we need to eat foods that resemble those our ancestors ate before the invention of factory-farmed meat and fish laden with chemicals, hormones, antibiotics, and pesticides. Our dietary requirements have been more than 2 million years in the making, but what we eat now looks nothing like the diet on which our primitive ancestors subsisted for millennia. And the amount of animal protein we eat today—North Americans consume ½ pound of meat a day, twice the world average—has grown exponentially since our ancestors were hunting and gathering.[38]

In short, many of us eat more protein than we need, even by the USDA's generous standard, which recommends ⅓ gram of protein per

Learn More

Want to learn more about pasture-based farming and meat? Check out this Web site: eatwild.com. Here, writers investigate the differences between animals raised in feedlots and those raised on pasture-based farms. The site, founded more than a decade ago, connects you with the pasture-based farm closest to your area and to farmers who will ship directly to you.

{Navigating the Landscape of Beef and Poultry Labels

Although labels increasingly read "grass-fed," "free-range," or "organic," these designations may be confusing at best to deceitful at worst. Here's a brief tutorial on what these terms really mean.[39]

Organic Beef. To be certified "organic," cattle must meet the following criteria:

- Born and raised on a certified organic pasture
- Never received antibiotics
- Never received growth-promoting hormones
- Fed only certified organic grains and grasses
- Had unrestricted outdoor access

Grass-Fed. This means that grass and forage were the feed sources for ruminant animals (such as cattle, sheep, bison, and llamas) for the duration of their lives after weaning. They can't be fed grain or grain by-products and must have continuous access to pasture during the growing season.

Free-Range or Free-Roaming. This term applies only to poultry raised for meat and means that the birds have been allowed some access to the outdoors, though it does not regulate how much time or the quality or size of the outdoor area. No other criteria, such as environmental quality, number of birds per enclosure, or amount of space per bird, need to be met to use this term.

There are no standards regarding the term "free-range" for egg-producing hens, although you might see the term on egg cartons. When they're used for eggs, free-range hens usually live uncaged in barns or warehouses, though they do have some outdoor access. There are no restrictions on what they're fed. Beak cutting and forced molting are permitted.

Cage-Free. This means that laying hens live in a barn or other enclosed area during their egg-production cycle. They're not confined to cages, are allowed to roam freely within their area, and they're given unlimited access to food and water. Outdoors access isn't required, and beak cutting is allowed.

Naturally Raised. This term refers to livestock raised without being fed growth hormones and antibiotics—except those needed to control parasites. Also, they are not fed by-products of animals or fish that have been harvested or slaughtered.

pound of body weight. So, for example, if you weigh 150 pounds, the USDA says you need about 50 grams of protein a day. If you weigh 180, you need about 60 grams. In general, women need 45 grams of protein each day; men need 56 grams. Just 3 ounces of meat—the size of a deck of cards—has about 21 grams of protein; an 8-ounce container of yogurt has about 11 grams; 1 cup of dry beans has about 16 grams. Added together, just these three sources would meet the protein needs of most women.

The LiverUp! Cleanse is plant centered. It is likely that you will be eating more plants—and a greater variety of plants—than you normally eat. The cleanse suggests eating as many leafy greens and veggies of every color as you can manage. It's just the first step toward mindful and healthy eating as a way to heal and strengthen your liver for the rest of your life. Longer term, you'll want to fill your plate with more plant and less animal protein—for your own health and for the health of the planet. Remember, it's not about deprivation, it's about feeding your body with the best fuel possible.

Some of you eat a plant-based diet only, while others eat fish and dairy. But most of you eat varying amounts of animal protein. No matter where you land on the spectrum, the LiverUp! Cleanse offers options to meet your needs. If you choose not to eat animal protein, there are many ways to get enough protein in vegetables and microalgae (page 118).

Let's look here at your many choices for healthy protein.

Beef. When it comes to animal protein, the science is in; Pastured, grass-fed beef is the healthier choice. The Union of Concerned Scientists reviewed and analyzed the scientific literature, comparing nutritional differences between pasture-raised, grass-fed cattle and conventionally raised (on grain in feed lots) cattle. Here's a summary of their findings.[40]

- Steak and ground beef from grass-fed cattle are almost always lower in total fat than steak and ground beef from conventionally raised cattle.

- Steak from grass-fed cattle tends to have higher levels of the omega-3 fatty acid ALA (alpha linolenic acid).

- Ground beef from grass-fed cattle contains higher levels of CLA (conjugated linolenic acid).

- Milk from pasture-raised cattle tends to have higher levels of ALA.

- Milk from pasture-raised cattle has consistently higher levels of CLA.

- Steak from grass-fed cattle sometimes has higher levels of omega-3 fatty acids.

The Mayo Clinic reports similar findings on grass-fed meat and wild game, adding that it may contain more antioxidants, which protect the body against heart disease and cancer.[41]

If you choose to eat meat, select only clean, grass-fed land animals. Conventional farming practices harm the environment and torture the animals, and meat from grain- or corn-fed livestock, including fish, can be high in toxins and omega-6 fats, all of which may contribute to inflammation-based diseases, such as heart disease, cancer, diabetes, obesity, and arthritis.

Fish. In general, fish is healthy and protein-rich. Some wild-caught fish, such as mackerel, sardines, and anchovies, are notable for their omega-3 fatty acids and their low level of contaminants. White-fleshed fish, such as cod, flounder, halibut, and rockfish, are leaner and thus provide less omega-3, but they still provide high-quality protein.

Wild salmon, an excellent source of protein, is also one of the best sources of omega-3 fatty acids. That's because wild salmon obtain all their omega-3s from the krill and shrimp they eat—that's what gives salmon their beautiful color and makes them rich in antioxidants.

Farm-raised salmon, however, are raised on grain (an unnatural diet for fish), are often dyed pink or orange, and are given antibiotics. They also contain a higher proportion of omega-6 fats. Choose wild over farm-raised whenever possible.

Sardines and anchovies are great choices. In addition to omega-3s, they're loaded with calcium and selenium, the trace mineral linked to lower rates of cancer. Since sardines and anchovies remain low on the food chain, they have fewer toxins, such as mercury. Enjoy anchovies in moderation; they're high in sodium.

Whey Protein Powder

If you choose to eat dairy, whey is an excellent source of protein. A by-product of milk and cheese, whey protein has been promoted for its health benefits since the time of the Greek physician Hippocrates.

High-quality whey protein, one of the richest food sources for maximizing glutathione in your body, also provides all the key amino acids for glutathione production. Remember that glutathione is one of the most powerful antioxidants in your body, supporting and protecting your immune system. Its main function is to protect both your cells and your mitochondria from oxidative stress and damage, destroying free radicals and helping your liver detox carcinogens.

Your body can't absorb and assimilate glutathione from supplements or food. Instead, it creates glutathione from amino acids. As you grow older, your body's ability to produce glutathione decreases because it produces fewer critical amino acids. So to maintain solid levels of glutathione, look to supplement your diet with amino acids found in cold-pressed whey protein powder that's derived from pasture-fed cows and is free of chemicals and sugar. Unless you have an allergy, sensitivity, or aversion to dairy, high-quality whey protein can help:

- Support your immune health

- Boost your energy

- Support your metabolism

- Support your beneficial gut bacteria

- Support your joint and muscle health

- Protect all your tissues' cells via its antioxidant properties

- Provide critical amino acids and proteins for overall optimal health

Vegetable Protein

There are a number of excellent plant-based sources of protein. Let's take a look at some of them.

Marine-based. Aquatic algae are considered to be both plant and animal species. As plants, they produce their own food; as animals, they eat other plants. Straddling these two kingdoms, microalgae offer unique nutritional advantages. First, they contain more chlorophyll than any other food. According to Paul Pitchford, a leading authority in nutrition and foundational healing and author of *Healing with Whole Foods,* chlorophyll has many healing properties, including the ability to:[42]

- Stop yeast and fungi growth in your digestive tract

- Remove toxic drug deposits and detoxify your body of heavy metals

- Neutralize many carcinogens

- Improve liver and intestinal function

- Reduce and perhaps even eliminate inflammation that causes sore throats, arthritis, and pancreatitis, among other conditions

- Reduce high blood pressure

These microorganisms also contain the highest concentrations of nucleic acids (RNA and DNA), protein, and beta-carotene found in any animal or plant food. Some studies suggest that nucleic acids may benefit cellular renewal and reverse aging.[43]

Microalgae also contain significant amounts of protein in a form

A Quick Guide to Plant Protein}

Nearly all vegetables, beans, grains, nuts, and seeds contain protein. As you'll see, it's easy to meet all of your protein requirements with vegetables. (For our cleanse, we'll be avoiding soy and legumes because of their challenge to our digestive system.)

FOOD	SERVING	PROTEIN (g)	PROTEIN (g/100 calories)
Tempeh	1 cup	31	9.6
Soybeans, cooked	1 cup	29	9.6
Lentils, cooked	1 cup	18	7.8
Black beans, cooked	1 cup	15	6.7
Kidney beans, cooked	1 cup	15	6.8
Chickpeas, cooked	1 cup	15	5.4
Pinto beans, cooked	1 cup	15	6.3
Lima beans, cooked	1 cup	15	6.8
Black-eyed peas, cooked	1 cup	13	6.7
Veggie baked beans	1 cup	12	5.0
Quinoa, cooked	1 cup	8	3.7
Peas, cooked	1 cup	8	6.6
Peanut butter	2 Tbsp	8	4.1
Almonds	¼ cup	8	3.7
Almond butter	2 Tbsp	7	3.4
Sunflower seeds	¼ cup	6	3.3
Cashews	¼ cup	5	2.7
Spinach, cooked	1 cup	5	13.0
Broccoli, cooked	1 cup	4	6.7

Source: USDA Nutrient Database for Standard Reference, release 24, 2011.

that's beneficial to those who eat an excessive amount of refined foods, sugar, and alcohol, plus significant amounts of animal protein—typically those who are overweight or who have diabetes, cancer, arthritis, or other diseases.[44] Much of the protein in microalgae, however, is in the form of biliprotein that has been predigested by the algae, making it easy for your body to digest and absorb.

Microalgae are diverse whole foods that help heal and restore balance for your body by:

- Strengthening and detoxing your body

- Reinforcing your immune system against invaders

- Increasing your body's energy

- Providing healing nourishment to help your body deal with stress and anxiety[45]

Hemp Seeds. We've already learned about the healing aspects of hemp seeds' omega-6 and omega-3 fatty acids, but they're also a great source of protein. These ancient seeds contain all of the essential amino acids, making them a complete plant protein. Three tablespoons of hemp seeds pack 11 grams of vegetable protein, making hemp a substantial source for those who choose to eat less animal protein.

Occasional Foods

Occasional foods are for those times when you're feeling a slight dip in energy or mood. Seeds, nuts, and nut butters will satisfy hunger pains and provide a bit of healthy plant fats. Sweet potatoes will help satisfy your sugar cravings.

Seeds, Nuts, and Nut Butters

Seeds and nuts provide healthy, plant-based fats—exactly the kind found in the Mediterranean Diet—shown in almost every study to be associated with lower levels of cardiovascular disease and cancer. Researchers at the Harvard School of Public Health combed through the Nurses' Health Study, the Iowa Women's Health Study, and the Adventist Health Study—three of the largest and most important long-term scientific studies—and concluded that people who eat nuts regularly are less likely to have a heart attack or to die from one. In fact, those who ate nuts several times a week had a 30 to 50 percent lower risk of heart attacks or heart disease than those who rarely or never consumed nuts.[46]

Along with healthy, monounsaturated fat, most nuts contain the amino acid arginine, which protects the inner lining of your arterial walls, making them more flexible and fluid and less susceptible to plaque buildup. Walnuts are the only nuts that contain omega-3 fatty acids, which your body can't make and which therefore must be obtained through your diet.

But be careful not to overeat nuts. Practice portion control—measure 1- or 2-ounce servings for snacks. As healthy as they are, too many at one sitting can overload your liver. They're included in your cleanse as a nutrient-dense snack that will keep your blood sugar levels even and balanced.

Sweet Potatoes

Sweet potatoes may seem like a surprising choice for a cleanse, but these starchy vegetables play an important role. When you set aside your favorite food "drugs," such as caffeine, sugar, processed carbs, and alcohol, you may feel a slight energy and mood dip for the first few days, as your body finds its equilibrium while it's detoxing from unhealthy foods.

This is when we turn to sweet potatoes. They're packed with calcium, potassium, and vitamins A, C, and E. Plus, they provide fiber and antioxidants, which help to eliminate free radicals, protecting your body from chemicals that damage cells, promote heart disease, and cause cancer. Sweet potatoes stabilize your blood sugar if you're feeling low in energy or mood. They contain an enzyme that contributes to their sugary flavor, yet because they contain high levels of fiber (almost twice as much fiber as other potatoes), their caloric energy is used more slowly and efficiently than low-fiber carbohydrates, keeping your blood sugar down and satisfying you longer. As a sweet-flavored snack or as part of a meal, sweet potatoes are a healthy, whole-food energy lifter.

In *Potatoes Not Prozac,* author Kathleen DesMaisons, PhD, asserts that sweet potatoes are particularly healing for those who suffer from sugar cravings, as they help your brain manufacture more serotonin, the chemical that lifts your mood and curbs cravings for sugar. Sweet potatoes work best in lifting serotonin levels if you eat them as a snack, several hours after a meal.[47] So if you're craving sweets or caffeine, or just feeling a bit sluggish—physically or emotionally—indulge in a sweet potato. It's a delicious, whole food–based pick-me-up.

Extra Support

Dandelion root tea and milk thistle supplement support your liver's Phase Two Detoxification Process. Dandelion root provides prebiotics and milk thistle supplies the powerful flavonoid, silymarin.

Dandelion Root Tea. You may remember that dandelion leaves support liver detoxification. And its roots contain inulin, a prebiotic that nourishes probiotics, those friendly bacteria in your gut.

Trying to come off coffee? Dandelion root tea makes a delicious substitute, with its earthy, robust flavor. It supports your intestinal flora, which play an essential role in detoxing your body. Other roasted herbs, like barley, can also make a nice morning tea.

Milk Thistle Supplement (200 milligrams). Milk thistle, a member of the sunflower family, has been used medicinally for more than 2,000 years. Its seeds contain silymarin, a flavonoid with antioxidant and anti-inflammatory properties.

Silymarin hunts for free radicals and inhibits their production. It protects your liver against toxins, including drugs such as acetaminophen (Tylenol), which can cause liver damage in high doses. Silymarin transforms the structure of liver cells so that toxins can't penetrate its organ walls.[48]

Studies suggest that milk thistle protects and supports your liver in a variety of ways: in its two-phase detoxification process, in increasing its speed to carry out its functions, and in both repairing injured liver cells and generating new ones that have been damaged by alcohol or other toxins. Milk thistle may also help reduce inflammation throughout your body.[49]

While milk thistle is available as a tea, its liver-supporting benefits decrease in water. It's most effective as a supplement combined with choline, which has been shown to help your body absorb milk thistle. Choline, a key element in cell membranes, helps silymarin attach easily to cell membranes, thus preventing toxins from getting inside liver cells.[50]

Milk thistle is generally regarded as safe with mild side effects, such as loose bowels that may last for 2 to 3 days. Also, it may interact with other herbs, supplements, or medications, so be sure to consult with your health-care provider before you begin taking it.

Foods to Avoid or Minimize

On the LiverUp! Cleanse, you have lots of delicious foods from which to choose. So you'll never go hungry. There are some foods you'll want to avoid as they sabotage your health and well-being.

Processed Foods, Refined Carbs, and Sugar

Remember that processed foods, which include white flour and sugar, are toxic to your liver and colon. Processed foods are laden with trans fats, processed or rancid fats, refined carbohydrates, chemicals, and toxins. Because of these additives, processed foods burden both phases of your liver's detoxification process, overload your digestive system, encourage yeast (candida), and inhibit probiotics and critical enzymes, interrupting your liver's ability to transform toxins.

Every refined carbohydrate calorie is either converted to glycogen in your muscles for future use or is eventually converted to triglycerides by your liver and stored as body fat. With a diet largely made up of refined foods, triglycerides will continue to increase, triggering cardiovascular disease, increased LDL (bad) cholesterol, atherosclerosis, and potential insulin resistance.

As if this weren't enough, the food industry has made an art of devising addictive products. In *Salt Sugar Fat: How the Food Giants Hooked Us,* author Michael Moss examines how food manufacturers have convinced consumers to ingest about twice the recommended amount of salt, some 70 pounds of sugar a year, and large quantities of trans fats in processed foods.[51]

While you may not be able to forgo every packaged food in your diet for the long haul, evidence shows that these "food products" are not

{Beware: Toxic Sweeteners

High-fructose corn syrup (HFCS) may be the most damaging sweetener to your health. Much like alcohol, fructose exacts a heavy toll on your liver, the only organ that can break it down. The result? Your body becomes a sea of toxic by-products. (By contrast, your liver has to break down only 20 percent of glucose, while the remaining 80 percent is immediately metabolized and used by the rest of your cells.)

As your body metabolizes HFCS, it creates fatty acids that build up as fat droplets in both your liver and your skeletal muscle tissues, which leads to insulin resistance and nonalcoholic fatty liver. Those conditions are precursors to metabolic syndrome and diabetes.

A study at the University of California, Davis, revealed that in just 10 weeks, a high-fructose diet can cause new fat cells to form around your heart, liver, and digestive organs, plunging you into the early stages of diabetes and heart disease.[52]

And HFCS and other sweeteners are hard to avoid. A study from the University of North Carolina shows that 80 percent of all food items are laced with added sugar.[53]

The bottom line: Avoid *all* processed foods and all of sugar's relatives—including high-fructose corn syrup (perhaps the most toxic of all). Be sure to read labels: Avoid molasses, sugar cane crystals, sugar cane juice, evaporated cane juice, maltodextrin, agave, and all products ending with "ose"—such as sucrose, fructose, dextrose, and levulose.

really food at all and should be avoided. During the cleanse, take them off the table.

Wheat and All Gluten-Containing Grains

Gluten is the key protein in wheat, rye, barley, some oats, and spelt. And for many of us, wheat—in the form of bread, pasta, pizza, crackers, cakes, or cookies—dominates our diets.

In 1985, the National Cholesterol Education Program advised us to eat more whole grains in place of fat and cholesterol. Since then, the Centers for Disease Control and Prevention (CDC) has been tracking body weight statistics. Their findings: There's been an upsurge in obesity and diabetes since that year.[54] As William Davis, MD, points out in *Wheat Belly*, the wheat we eat today is very different than *einkorn*, the wheat our ancestors ate thousands of years ago.[55] Today, *einkorn* and other wild and cultivated strains of wheat have been replaced by a variety called *Triticum*, a higher-yielding, more disease-, drought-, and heat-resistant variety. It's hybridized and genetically modified—and it's harming our health.[56]

✘ Whole wheat bread increases blood sugar more quickly—and to higher levels—than sucrose, triggering a surge in insulin, which in turn converts blood glucose into fat around your abdomen, creating a "wheat belly." The more wheat products you consume, the higher and more frequently your blood glucose spikes, and the more insulin you produce. With sustained production of insulin (the hormone that allows glucose to enter your cells and converts this glucose to fat), your tissues eventually become resistant to insulin. When this happens, your liver loses its insulin sensitivity. It can't interpret signals properly and begins to convert stored glycogen to blood sugar, which raises blood sugar levels even further. This puts more pressure on your pancreas to secrete even more insulin. Thus the process feeds upon itself.

Meanwhile, you begin to experience carb and sugar cravings, along with mood swings, flagging energy, and an inability to focus. An increased consumption of these grains—coupled with a decreased consumption of healthy fats—has made us sick. We've also learned that foods your body can't digest pass through your intestinal wall and are treated as toxins in your bloodstream.

And since your digestive tract is where detoxification begins, the more foods that seep through your gut wall, the harder your liver must work, targeting these new toxins rather than focusing on toxins already present in your body. For many of us, gluten is one such toxin, signaling your immune system to kick into overdrive and further burdening your liver.

Dairy

Avoid most conventionally produced dairy products. Cow's milk tops the list of the most common food allergies because once we're weaned as children, many of us stop producing lactase, the enzyme that digests milk sugar, or lactose. Without lactase, we become lactose intolerant, experiencing digestive upset—stomach cramps, gas, bloating, even diarrhea—when we eat dairy products. These symptoms increase gut permeability, placing a greater load on your liver.

Plus, many people have an allergy to casein, a milk protein, and that allergy causes the immune system to treat dairy as a toxic invader (a pathogen), triggering antibodies that kick-start the liver into targeting it. When the liver must work at transforming, neutralizing, and detoxing the invading pathogen, it becomes burdened and can't perform some of its critical tasks, such as completing its two-phase detoxification, metabolizing fat, and producing adequate amounts of bile, all of which rid your body of toxins already present.

And nonorganic milk can contain traces of hormones and antibiotics given to feedlot cattle, plus pesticides and fertilizer residues in their food. Raw, organic, pasture-fed butter, however, can be a rich source of beneficial nutrients, including vitamin A and selenium.

Trans Fats

Trans fats are man-made fats found in margarine, vegetable shortening, vegetable oils—including canola and soybean oils—and nearly all fast foods, most processed foods, and most commercial baked goods, chips, and crackers. These fats are valuable to commercial food manufacturers because they extend the shelf life of every packaged food, but they wreak havoc on your health and well-being.

Almost every packaged food contains hydrogenated or partially hydrogenated oils—even those claiming to be trans fat free—because a loophole in the law allows a certain amount of trans fats per serving before the product manufacturer must disclose that the food contains them.

Dr. Mary Enig, a renowned biochemist and nutritionist best known for her pioneering work on healthy fats and her protest against the use of trans fats decades ago, has done some of the most important research on this topic. In *Eat Fat, Lose Fat,* Dr. Enig asserts that trans fats:

- Lower HDL (good) cholesterol

- Raise LDL (bad) cholesterol

- Increase blood insulin levels

- Cause tissues to lose omega-3 fatty acids

- Interfere with many enzyme functions and with the immune system[57]

The bottom line: These oils burden your liver and can lead to cardiovascular disease, diabetes, and cancer. Read labels carefully. Avoid commercial canola or soybean oils and any products made with these oils—tortilla and potato chips, crackers, baked goods, commercial breads, microwave popcorn, and fried and fast foods.

Caffeine and Alcohol

Your body treats both caffeine and alcohol as toxins, which stress your liver and fatigue its efforts to metabolize fat and rid your body of toxins. Plus, as a diuretic, caffeine is dehydrating, encouraging your body to rid itself of fluids—even though your body needs a lot of water to flush itself of toxins.

Caffeine works a lot like sugar. After ingesting it, you may experience an initial lift in energy and mood, only to feel a bit sluggish, weak, and lethargic after the initial buzz wears off. With caffeine, your body ends up with more adrenaline coursing through its veins. That can make you feel alert, motivated, and stimulated. For some of us, though, the extra adrenaline can make us feel jittery and anxious.

When you consume caffeine and these stimulants flood your body, it acts to protect itself by shutting down receptors for dopamine and adrenaline—which means you end up needing more adrenaline, feeling more fatigued, and craving more caffeine. Caffeine, particularly coffee, is one of the most difficult substances to give up. If you take on this challenge, you may experience some tough withdrawal symptoms at first: headache, cravings, irritability, fatigue, depression, anxiety, nervousness, and lack of focus. These are totally normal and last only a day or two.

To help you come off caffeine, vitamin C is helpful. You'll be consuming lots of it in the fruits and vegetables recommended for your cleanse. Vitamin C supports your adrenal glands, which are stressed by the highs and lows of caffeine consumption. These glands will help you during withdrawal, as well.

The most important task during cleanse days will be to drink half your body weight in ounces of water to flush the caffeine out of your body. You can ease your way into a caffeine-free cleanse one step at a time. Try taking your coffee or other caffeinated beverages as a mixture of half caffeinated, half decaf for several days, or limit your caffeine intake by half for a few days. Or you may want to go cold turkey. Listen to your body. It'll tell you what it needs to free itself of caffeine for 12 days.

Alcohol. Your liver considers alcohol to be even more toxic than caffeine because alcohol taxes both your liver and your gut. The more alcohol you consume, the more antioxidants you need. That's because to detox alcohol, your liver requires an enzyme dependent on a full supply of antioxidants, especially vitamin C.

Before alcohol travels to your liver, it lands in your gut, where it acts like an intestinal irritant, increasing the risk of intestinal permeability, disrupting healthy intestinal bacteria, and disturbing digestion and nutrient absorption. As a result, you may experience a deficiency in various nutrients and vitamins, especially the B vitamins, vitamin C, magnesium, and zinc.

To support your liver in detoxing your body of existing toxins, limit additional toxins during your cleanse. Consider replacing your cocktail or glass of wine with:

- Water with a few frozen berries tossed in

- Lemon water

- Mineral water with a splash of pure pomegranate juice

Soy Products

Soy is found in processed soy foods, such as soy milk, soy cheese, soy ice cream, soy hot dogs, soy burgers, tofu, and any unfermented soy product, as well as low-carbohydrate energy bars and soy protein powders. Unprocessed soy (soybeans) can be packaged as edamame or as crunchy soybean nuts.

Soybeans contain more phytic acid than any other grain or legume. These high levels reduce your body's ability to absorb or assimilate important minerals, such as calcium, magnesium, copper, iron, and zinc. In soy, phytic acid isn't neutralized by soaking, sprouting, or slow cooking, as it is in various grains.

While studies linking soy to cancer are conflicting and inconclusive, Cornell University's Program on Breast Cancer and Environmental Risk Factors concludes that "both animal and human studies suggest that soy phytoestrogens can behave like estrogen and potentially increase breast cancer risk. Some scientists have suggested that women should be cautious about eating large amounts of the soy products or soy supplements, because of the possible harmful effects of soy phytoestrogens."[58]

One of the ways higher estrogen exposure may be linked to breast cancer risk is through its ability to increase growth of milk ducts, where most breast cancer arises. Several studies examining the effect of soy phytoestrogens on breast growth in women have suggested that phytoestrogens have a weak estrogen-like effect. One such study tracked 29 women who took a soy supplement for 6 months. While they were taking the supplement, their milk ducts grew, potentially increasing their risk for breast cancer.[59]

Since there may be evidence linking soy to damaging health conditions, for the purposes of your cleanse, I recommend forgoing it for at least 12 days, and perhaps forever.

All Sweeteners—Except Stevia

Stevia is an herbal sweetener derived from a South American plant. Besides its sweetness, studies have shown that stevia may have a number of health benefits: It may lower blood sugar and blood pressure. Stevia may also have antidiarrheal and anti-inflammatory properties. It could help regulate your immune system.[60]

Stevia comes in both liquid and granule forms. It's best to consume stevia in its most unrefined form—in a dark liquid tincture. Several brands, including SweetLeaf and Stevita, come in tinctures or granules that are unrefined.

Suggestions—Not Straitjackets

These foods are suggested guidelines for your 12-day cleanse. But every person is unique. Your physical, emotional, mental, and spiritual makeup is completely individual, so the way you need to fuel your body, tend to your mind, and nurture your spirit will be unique, too. So honor your own individuality and choose foods that work for you.

Anyone can do the LiverUp! Cleanse, anywhere, any time. It's a simple eating program to satisfy everyone from omnivores to vegans. You may find that some of these foods don't appeal to you. That's okay. There are plenty of foods from which to choose: dark leafy greens, a cornucopia of vegetables, colorful berries, warming spices, cleansing herbs, satiating fats, protein from both animal and plant sources, and lots of water. Fortifying for your liver and cleansing for your colon, these foods aid in detoxifying your entire system, while energizing and rejuvenating your mind, body, and spirit.

Remember: This cleanse isn't an exercise in deprivation—you may find it challenging to eat as many vegetables as recommended, so take it slow. Take a few days to ease into it. Turn to the menus in the Appendix to help guide you day by day.

In the next chapter, you'll learn about the optional fast that can be part of your cleanse. Read Chapter 6 to decide whether a fast is right for you. The gift of cleansing is that it will help you hear what your body tells you and will give you the tools to respond in a gentle, loving, and self-compassionate way.

SUSAN EHRHARD, 54

Living Mindfully

Lost: 9 pounds

Menopause middle: Shrunk

Skin: Clear

Energy: Increased

Over the last few years, I'd put on 20 extra pounds and it's easy to see how. I work in an office all day and I can't work out the way I used to because I have arthritis in my knees. Every night after work, I'd have a drink, then munch on sweets in bed while I watched the evening news. I found I was eating lots of breads, lots of pasta, and way too many sweets. But though the pounds were creeping on and my clothes weren't fitting anymore, I didn't really care what I looked like. I knew I needed to do something, but I wasn't sure what. I was in a place I couldn't get out of and I didn't have the energy or the willpower to start another "diet."

But the cleanse made all the difference. The mantra, "Be mindful of what you eat," was exactly what I needed. I learned about new greens to use into my salads, and I loved the kale smoothies. I liked the fact that I could load up on the greens, add fresh vegetables, and then add protein, such as chicken. The recipes satisfied my hunger and were delicious, especially with the addition of flax seeds and hemp protein powder. And an apple before bedtime was the perfect end to my day—of course I ate it in bed while watching the news!

I know the LiverUp! Cleanse isn't a diet, but I've lost 9 pounds. My skin looks better, I feel better, and my menopause middle has gone down. I haven't had one drop of alcohol since the start of the cleanse, and my energy level at night is so much greater. I've been sleeping through the night and waking up feeling refreshed, energetic, and just plain awesome.

Although I've gone back to my 2 cups of coffee in the morning, I don't plan to start drinking alcohol every night. I realize that if I want to be the best I can be, I need to be mindful about all my choices.

CHAPTER 6

The LiverUp! Short-Term Fast

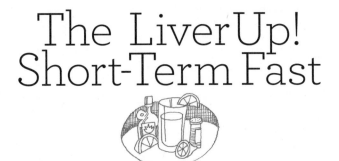

Now that you've learned about the foods you'll be enjoying on the LiverUp! Cleanse, let's look at the optional 1- to 2-day fast that takes place right after the 8th day of the cleanse. So if you begin cleansing on a Monday and you choose to fast, you'll start on the following Tuesday. Remember: Fasting is completely optional.

While fasting is healing for many, helping to prevent physical degeneration by eliminating toxic buildup in tissues and organs, allowing organs and systems to rest, and rebuilding cells, it's not for everyone. **It's always best to check with your doctor before taking on any type of fast, particularly if you have preexisting health conditions.**

Fasting gives your body a break from consuming, digesting, and assimilating food. The variations on fasting are endless. Some regimens require you to skip breakfast; others, dinner. Some require you to fast all day once a week, once a month, or even once a season.

Traditionally, fasting has meant abstaining from solid food and replacing it with lots of hydration—water or juices from fresh fruits and vegetables, along with herbal teas. But some practitioners consider fasts to include limited foods, such as raw fruits, raw vegetables, steamed vegetables, or rice-based porridges cooked with plenty of water, like kitchari or congee (see Chapter 9 for recipes). For our purposes, fasting means no solid food and lots of hydration for a short period of time—1 or 2 days max.

Fasting: A Path to Physical and Spiritual Well-Being

The practice of fasting is part of our evolutionary history. Over the many millennia that humans have inhabited the earth, our food supply has waxed and waned. We evolved by taking advantage of this ebb and flow, building muscle and fatty tissue during times of abundance, paring back during leaner times.

Over the centuries, fasting has been used as a means of healing—physically, emotionally, and spiritually. Yoga practices that include fasting date back thousands of years. Paramahansa Yogananda, a renowned Indian yogi who introduced Westerners to the practice of fasting in the 20th century, held that fasting is a natural method of healing.[1] Even today, the ancient healing practice of Ayurveda—the 5,000-year-old system of natural healing originating in India—includes fasting as therapy. Its most traditional method of fasting uses kitchari, a dish of rice and beans cooked with lots and lots of water.

In our Western tradition, the Bible refers to fasting, too. Moses, Elijah, and Jesus fasted for 40 days, a time of purification and enlightenment. The Essenes, the Jewish group that authored the Dead Sea Scrolls, wrote in one of their 3rd-century BCE manuscripts: "Seek the angel of fresh air, the angel of water, the angel of sunlight, and the angel of the earth, and invite them to stay with you throughout the fast!"[2] A wide variety of spiritual traditions have incorporated fasting into their practices.

Early Greek philosophers and healers used fasting as therapy. Paracelsus and Hippocrates, fathers of Western medicine, were both proponents of fasting. "Fasting is the greatest remedy—the physician within," wrote Paracelsus, while Hippocrates insisted that "to eat when you are sick is to feed your sickness."

Aligning with Nature's Rhythms

Fasting aligns us with nature as our bodies move with the cycles of life. From time to time, our cells need to fall like leaves from the trees before they can regenerate and be renewed. This process is called autophagy, and we'll discuss it further on page 140.

Traditional Chinese medicine practitioners argue that we experience disease when we don't live in accord with nature. We know that this is true when it comes to nature's food supply; it is much healthier than foods made in a laboratory. And consider your own sleep patterns. Is it easier to rise early when the sun comes up at 5 a.m. in June or when it rises at 7 a.m. in December? Think about the foods you prefer in the summer. At that time of year, you'd probably choose a lunch of fresh garden vegetables over a steaming plate of macaroni and cheese.

As we align ourselves with nature, fasting may be the best natural healing therapy for some of us. After all, nature provides a precedent: Instinctually, animals fast when they're stressed or ill. While we humans might resist the idea, it can be a beneficial way to experience balance, as we pause and come back to the things that are most important in our lives.

Traditional Chinese medicine follows nature by providing transitional times for cleansing and fasting—as winter moves into spring and as summer moves into fall. And in the West, people often yearn to cleanse after the winter holidays. Your cleanse will help you determine the right time to fast, as you connect with your body in a profound way. When you find balance by feeding your body with healing foods and practicing self-care, you will know, intuitively, whether fasting is the right action for you at this time. If you feel it's right, go for it. If you don't, perhaps you'll want to try it another time. The key is to honor what you hear your body telling you. Again, an important word of caution: A qualified health practitioner can guide and supervise your decision. (Note that fasting is not ideal in colder weather, when your body tends to want warmth.)

Just like cleansing, the gift that short-term fasting offers is space and time to listen to your body. Make an intention to discern your body's voice and honor it, whether it tells you to carry on with your cleanse or take an optional 1- or 2-day fast.

The Western Practice of Fasting

Many of us in developed countries suffer from the consequences of over-indulgence in foods laden with unhealthy fats, excess sugar, and chemicals that produce increased acids. These lead to weight gain and inflammatory degenerative diseases such as diabetes, heart disease, atherosclerosis, and hypertension. In a place with so many natural resources, it's astonishing that more and more North Americans are overfed and undernourished, experiencing a continuum of disease that's worsening daily. But many progressive physicians, researchers, and health educators recognize the importance of healing the body with clean, whole food—and less of it.

Herbert Shelton, ND (1895–1985), one of the earliest influential voices on cleansing and fasting, wrote 40 books during his 60-year career in health education. He supervised more than 40,000 fasts of chronically ill and terminal patients. Shelton's teachings on fasting inspired Indian peace activist Mahatma Gandhi, as well as contemporary physicians and health practitioners.

Shelton believed that the best action to take when first becoming ill is to stop eating and rest—contrary to the prevailing advice then (and now) to take a drug, eat to keep up your strength, and keep on going. In *Fasting Can Save Your Life,* Shelton presents the body as a self-healing organism and cleansing or fasting as the remedy that allows it the space to heal itself. Improper or excessive food, he insists, thwarts the natural ongoing healing processes.

Shelton believed that when we're sick, it's often best to fast. Rather than starving your body of essential nutrition, short-term fasting allows for conservation of the energy that would've been spent in digestion so that energy can be used to repair tissues, eliminate toxins, and fight disease. Remember: For the LiverUp! Cleanse, fasting means drinking highly nutritious juices—not just water—while taking a break from solid foods.

Healers and physicians with a holistic or spiritual orientation have been recommending fasting for decades. Elson Haas, MD; Joel Fuhrman, MD; Gabriel Cousens, MD; James Balch, MD; and Paul Pitchford are among the prominent contemporary proponents of fasting.

The Science behind the Practice

More and more, science is confirming that fasting benefits the body and mind. Let's take a look at some of the recent findings.

Fasting Slows the Aging Process

Scientists at the National Institute on Aging, led by Mark Mattson, professor of neuroscience at the Johns Hopkins University School of Medicine, have proven that fasting twice a week can significantly lower your risk of developing Alzheimer's and Parkinson's disease.[3] One of the only ways to slow the progression of aging that leads to disease or organ malfunction, they determined, is to reduce energy intake. These findings confirm decades-old studies revealing a link between caloric intake and oxidative cell deterioration or "rusting"—the stress on cells that comes when we age and consume more food than our bodies need.

Your brain and muscles, Mattson insists, benefit from being mildly stressed. One way to accomplish that: occasional, or intermittent, fasting, which revs up cellular defenses against molecular damage. "Our ancestors undoubtedly had to go without food for stretches of time," Mattson explains. "It hasn't been that long since humanity lacked regular supplies of food. When you search for food when you're hungry, the brain is really engaged. The individuals who survive the best—the ones whose brains are more attuned to predators and who can remember where food sources are—are the ones who've survived."[4]

Michael Mosley, a British physician and medical journalist, also researched intermittent fasting for his BBC documentary *Eat, Fast, and Live Longer.*[5] His conclusion: Mild hunger can trigger your body—and brain—to repair itself. Among the scientists whose work he examined was Krista Varady, PhD, of the University of Illinois at Chicago. In one of her studies, 32 overweight middle-aged volunteers with a median age of 42 were put on an alternate-day intermittent fast. At the end of 8 weeks, they'd lost an average of 9 pounds and seen significant improvements in biomarkers related to the risks of diabetes and coronary heart disease.[6]

A recent study at the Salk Institute for Biological Studies showed that mice that feasted on fatty foods for 8 hours a day and subsequently fasted for the rest of each day did not become obese or show dangerously high insulin levels. The study's senior researcher writes: "Our findings suggest that regular eating times and fasting for a significant number of hours a day may well be beneficial to our health."[7] This research also suggests that *when* we eat may be as important as *what* we eat. Giving your liver a break from eating allows this vital organ to protect your body from packing on the pounds, while lowering your risk of many metabolic diseases, including diabetes.

How come? Turns out it's all about the mitochondria in your liver, which process food in alternating cycles of work and rest. The mitochondria—your cell's powerhouses—divide while they're resting, so eating makes them work when they should be resting—and this unsettles the normal cycle, causing more DNA damage compared to mitochondria that are allowed to rest and divide in peace. In the Salk study, mice that ate for 8 hours and stopped eating for 10- to 12-hour stretches made more efficient use of their nutrients and ended up with more energy than the other mice. According to researchers, the mice who ate for just 8 hours were "protected against obesity, hyperinsulinemia, fatty liver disease, inflammation, and had improved motor coordination."[8]

These researchers found that the liver doesn't adhere to our circadian rhythms. While our internal clock separates functions throughout the day so our organs can stay healthy, the liver's clock doesn't monitor light and darkness to organize its functions based on the time of day. Instead, says the study, your liver's clock is set by your eating schedule: When you've eaten your last bite for a long span of time, your liver knows it's safe for its mitochondria to divide. This usually happens at the end of the day.[9] But if you're eating all the time, your liver's clock gets triggered too often. It repeatedly tries to adjust and, as one author stated, "it never knows when it's breakfast."[10] This is probably why shift workers experience much higher rates of metabolic disease than those who work according to more standard daytime schedules.

Research shows that your liver functions at its best when you give yourself a break from sabotaging foods that make it work overtime. Western science is beginning to prove what Eastern medicine has held as truth for centuries: There is unseen energy being directed through your body that naturally inclines it toward balance, healing, and health. Your body is marvelously miraculous at healing itself. Your job is to nurture and nourish it so it can do its job. Short-term fasting is one way to do this. Here are some ways it works to improve your well-being.

Fasting Kick-Starts Cellular Autophagy

Short-term fasting accelerates your body's process of clearing out waste left by dead and damaged cells in a process called autophagy[11]—a critical garbage-collecting and recycling process in healthy cells. As we get older, the process slows down, allowing toxins and waste to accumulate in cells, damaging parts of cells and tissues, and contributing to—or even defining—the process of aging.

But short-term fasting enables each cell to flush itself of stored and circulating toxins. Recent research at Children's Hospital Los Angeles showed that fasting cleanses your blood and your lymph systems so that they can eliminate those toxins released by cells and tissues. With fewer metabolic demands, cells can repair themselves as they rid themselves of waste. Perhaps most importantly, your liver, colon, kidneys, sinuses, and skin can focus on detoxifying your body rather than targeting new, incoming chemicals as these organs process and discharge stored toxins.[12]

Brain health depends on autophagy of neurons—the brain cells that send impulses to every part of your body. The Children's Hospital study shows that when an "essential autophagy gene" in the neurons of fetal mice is removed, the result is more body fat, poor glucose tolerance, and impaired nervous system development.[13] Without the process of autophagy, your brain can't develop properly or work well.

So giving your body time and space for autophagy is critical, and that's what happens during the process of detoxification and fasting. The first couple of days of your cleanse can be challenging if your diet has included sugar, wheat, coffee, and alcohol—that can be a lot to give up all at one time. If you stay with it, though, your body will flush those stored toxins out, and you'll feel a sense of lightness and ease within a couple of days.

While everyone experiences fasting differently, there are shared metabolic commonalities. When your body releases stored toxins, your cells experience increased oxygenation, improved functionality, and rejuvenation.

In *Fasting and Eating for Health,* Joel Fuhrman, MD, explains the process this way:

> Therapeutic fasting is not a mystical or magical cure. It works because the body has within it the capacity to heal when the obstacles to healing are removed. Health is the normal state. Most chronic disease is the inevitable consequence of living a life-style that places disease-causing stressors on the human organism. Fasting gives the body an interlude without those stressors so that it can speedily repair or accomplish healing that could not otherwise occur in the feeding state.[14]

Fasting Strengthens Your Liver to Help Your Body Resist Disease

Your liver is your most overworked organ, and your diet requires it to work relentlessly, resulting in ongoing fatigue. Giving your liver a break from this unremitting job allows it to metabolize existing toxins and eliminate them from your body. Mattson and others have confirmed that short-term, intermittent fasting strengthens your liver in "affecting energy, oxygen radical metabolism, and cellular stress response systems, in ways that protect neurons against genetic and environmental factors to which they would otherwise succumb during aging."[15] In other words, Mattson says, fasting "helps cells cope with stress and resist disease."[16]

Fasting Flushes Your Body of Acidic Congestion

Fasting is beneficial for those who suffer from acidic congestive conditions, such as colds, flu, sinusitis, arthritis, atherosclerosis, diabetes, sluggish digestion, and fatigue. Your body strives to maintain a pH balance in your blood between 7.3 and 7.5, the pH range in which your metabolism, enzymes, and immune system work most effectively. Since your body is sensitive to blood pH levels, it works constantly to maintain homeostasis, or balance. When you continually consume acid-producing foods—sugars, chemicals, and the unhealthy fats contained in processed foods—your body seeks sodium and potassium (mainly an intracellular mineral) to neutralize your blood. These minerals are stored outside your cells in extracellular fluid. When these extracellular stores are depleted, your body goes looking for calcium, magnesium, and other alkalizing minerals from your bones and other sources, as well. Additionally, some acidity results from excess phosphorus and sulfur from too much protein, and this can cause calcium to be pulled from bones and tissues.

Your cells react negatively to an internal acidic condition by becoming sluggish and unable to function properly. Waste builds up, toxins are stored, nutrients aren't properly assimilated, and you become sick. According to Russell M. Jaffe, MD, a diet that consists of excess acids—and results in low levels of potassium and magnesium—can lead to toxin accumulation. "A number of large research studies involving thousands of participants," he writes, "have reported about the association between metabolic acidosis and insulin resistance, type 2 diabetes, cardio-metabolic risk, coronary heart disease, and osteoporosis. A typical American diet provides insufficient minerals and fiber to counter or buffer the buildup of metabolic acids and to help displacement of toxic wastes." He goes on to say that the body's ability to produce energy and safely remove toxins is compromised when even minor increases in acidity occur. Metabolic acidosis has also been linked to chronic fatigue immune dysfunction syndrome. In his medical practice, Jaffe has observed "restoration of vitality and quality of life when metabolic acidosis is corrected comprehensively."[17] Jaffe's recommendation: a nutrient-rich alkaline diet of whole foods from locally grown, vine-ripened, organic sources, plus mineral-rich water.

Cleansing or fasting with large amounts of alkalizing foods, water, or water-based juices allows your body to flush out acidic metabolites and toxins that can cause disease, while simultaneously strengthening your immune system. According to Jaffe, the optimal diet is high in fresh fruits and vegetables, a few whole grains, and small amounts of protein—essentially an alkalizing diet. Plus, quality whey protein—including that from grass-fed cows—provides essential amino acids such as glutamine and cysteine, along with fatty acids such as conjugated linoleic acid. As we've learned, high cysteine levels hugely support glutathione levels and, thus, antioxidant function.

Fasting Promotes Weight Loss

Depending on the number of calories in what you drink while fasting, fasting reduces caloric intake, requiring your liver to convert stored glycogen into glucose, and thus, energy. This process, called gluconeogenesis, initiates weight loss. Here's how it works.

While much of your body can use its own fat for energy, your brain, central nervous system, and red blood cells need glucose. When you fast, your glycogen stores diminish as your liver is required to convert its stored glycogen back into glucose and release it into your bloodstream. If fasting continues, the stores of glycogen in your liver become depleted, and your body turns to its stored fat to convert that into fatty acids and then into glucose.

When your body needs to raid your fat cells for glucose stores, insulin regulates how much fat gets converted to fatty acids and then transports these fatty acids around your body to your cells. Once it reaches your cells, your insulin releases the fatty acids, which are then converted into glucose for energy.

When you fast or abstain from processed foods, refined carbohydrates, and sugars, your body goes looking for glucose in your fat cells, begins to burn its own fuel, and starts dropping weight.[18]

Fasting Provides Mental, Emotional, and Spiritual Benefits

As scientists study the effects of short-term fasting on both mice and humans, they're beginning to gather data proving that detoxing and fasting lead to better health. Until recently, it's been difficult to study the multidimensional process of detoxing and fasting in comparison with a different diet or placebo. The double-blind, placebo-controlled gold standard of research is much easier when only one substance is being controlled—for example, high-fructose corn syrup or a new drug. Some of the best data we have is from those who have participated in a period of detoxification and reported increased energy, clarity, improved concentration, more restful sleep, and an overall feeling of well-being.

The process of eliminating substances and simplifying your intake for short periods of time allows you to listen and learn how your body responds. Knowing what works for you—and what doesn't—takes your healing from an intellectual exercise to one that you experience in your body and heart, making it easier to put this knowledge into practice.

When you commit to detoxing your body, you engage in your own healing as you openly embrace a process of transformation. As your body eliminates dead matter (autophagy) and releases stored toxins, allowing your cells to rejuvenate, you experience a renewed sense of clarity and energy, allowing you to live in the present moment and remain open to the future. Detoxification can refer to anything that you let go. The process of abstaining from food allows you to let go of those mental and emotional attachments that keep you stuck, often paralyzing you in a pattern of sabotaging behavior.

Detoxification allows you the space and time to dislodge repressed feelings and genuinely experience them—anger, resentments, hurt, fear. When you're willing to feel your feelings, often you can welcome them and work through them with joy, love, and forgiveness, freeing your body, mind, and spirit to heal. Gentle, graceful shifts in the way you eat, over time, lead to significant shifts in your life toward health and wholeness.

Elson Haas, MD, has been using the process of detoxification for more than 35 years and has supervised thousands of patients in cleansing and fasting. In *Staying Healthy with Nutrition,* he writes about the mental and emotional benefits of detoxing via cleansing and fasting.

> . . . fasting (and detoxification) is the missing link in the American (and Western) diet. . . . Taking breaks from things is a good way to assess our true relationship to them and often a way to improve our health. When we treat ourselves with more respect and generate an attitude of self-love, of caring for the body in a positive and loving way, we will choose less polluting ways of living, and this lifestyle will produce less personal and planetary toxicity.[19]

For Haas, cleansing and fasting are vehicles to freedom from addiction of all kinds. "It helps us to open to our true guidance, growth, potentials, and life. Fasting opens us spiritually and emotionally, and supports us in becoming more real in our lives, in doing what we believe and know in our hearts and spirits to be right for us."[20]

Gabriel Cousens, MD, has also written extensively on the mental and spiritual benefits of fasting.

> Spiritual fasting helps people to discover their holy rhythm and to align with the rhythm of the living earth and universe. . . . This 5,000-year-old approach still seems the

most fundamental, elegantly simplistic, and profound in helping people access the deep healing force than anything else we have. The body is self-cleansing, self-healing, and self-regenerating.[21]

The Nuts and Bolts of Fasting

There are many ways to fast. The key is to listen to your body and connect with your intuition. Both will tell you what's appropriate for you now—this time in your life, the season of the year, the day of the week. Part of the healing process is how you respond. Be sure you're fasting in a self-loving, healing way rather than as a means of punishment or deprivation.

Careful preparation is key. A sensible plan begins with first detoxing the body for a period of time.

The LiverUp! 12-day Cleanse eliminates many toxins, chemicals, sugars, and acid-producing foods, replacing them with alkaline-based foods: dark leafy greens, multicolored vegetables, berries, sea vegetables, prebiotic- and probiotic-rich foods, small amounts of clean protein, and lots of water. Plus, the cleanse fuels your body with a high-nutrient, low-toxin diet, fortifying your liver, flushing your cells and tissues, and strengthening your body in preparation for a fast.

To prepare your mind and body for a short-term fast, as you make your way through the cleanse, begin to commit to fasting from after dinner until breakfast. You may want to take a day or two and only eat fruits and vegetables to further detox your body and ease the transition before fasting.

Each fasting protocol has its own benefits. We'll consider a few here, but if none of these protocols meet your needs, this may not be the time for you to fast. If that's the case, simply carry on with your cleanse. The LiverUp! Cleanse is a way of eating that you can embrace for a lifetime. That's because there's no limit to how long you can cleanse, as long as you have a balanced diet that contains all of your needed nutrients. Our cleanse involves eating a broad variety of beautiful vegetables, berries, sea vegetables, a limited amount of clean protein, healthy fats, and plenty of water.

Fasting Option #1: Fresh Vegetable and Fruit Juice Fast

Vegetable and fruit juice fasting is a mild and effective technique used by many practitioners and fasting clinics. As almost every health practitioner recommends consuming 6 to 8 servings of vegetables and fruits per day, juicing is an easy way to guarantee that you'll get necessary amounts of these vital nutrients. Fresh juices from raw vegetables and fruits are easily assimilated and require minimum digestion, allowing you to absorb all of the nutrients. Juices provide the benefits of raw foods without the complications of digesting so much fiber, since much of the fiber in juice is discarded.

The Science Behind Juicing

Juicing allows you to consume more vegetables and more parts of a plant than you'd ordinarily eat, providing you with a wide range of nutrients. Your body can absorb nutrient-dense juice almost instantly, requiring little effort. It is like giving yourself an infusion of vitamins, minerals, and enzymes that goes right into your system for immediate energy. Raw vegetable and fruit juices supply calories, vital phytonutrients, vitamins, minerals, and essential enzymes (many of which are killed by cooking). Some advocates suggest "chewing your juice." "Chew your juice and juice your food" is one of the philosophies of natural hygiene.

Recent studies have confirmed several benefits of juicing. In a study at Kings College London and other British institutions, participants who'd been diagnosed with hypertension and who were not taking any medication for the condition were divided into two groups. Half were asked to drink 20 ounces of beetroot juice; the others were instructed to simply drink the same amount of water. Those who drank the juice showed significant decreases in their blood pressure readings.[22]

And researchers at the Vanderbilt University School of Medicine, in a study involving nearly 2,000 participants, found that fruits and vegetables may play an important role in delaying the onset of Alzheimer's disease. People who drank freshly made fruit and vegetable juices more than three times per week, compared to those who did so less than once a week, were 76 percent less likely to develop Alzheimer's disease.[23]

Typically, juices are made from a variety of vegetables and fruits. Dark leafy greens and apples with lemon and ginger are warming and enhance digestion, according to Ayurvedic medicine, while a combination of spinach, carrots, celery, and lemon is cleansing and energizing.

Vegetable juices (with or without fresh fruit) can be consumed all

{Some Juicing Caveats

- Use the freshest, most chemical-free fruits and vegetables possible. Organic, local, and seasonal are your best options. If your ingredients aren't organic, they should be peeled.
- Juicing requires special equipment, although several relatively inexpensive juicers are available. Be sure to follow the directions on your juicer for optimum results.
- Fresh juices are also available at health food stores, juice bars, and raw food eateries.
- Some juices don't hold up well in oxygen and sunlight; they can oxidize or break down. Drink freshly made juices almost immediately so the nutrients aren't exposed to the elements. Some vitamins and phytonutrients, such as vitamin C, carotenoids, and bioflavonoids, oxidize and diminish within minutes.
- If you don't care for straight vegetable juices, add some fruit juice, but remember that the extracted juices from most fruits are high in fructose or fruit sugar. While they contain calories, and thus energy, along with some vitamins and minerals, too much fructose can be a burden on your liver (as well as your pancreas and your adrenal gland) so keep fruit sugars low, particularly when consuming them without the fiber of the whole fruit.

day, for breakfast, lunch, and dinner, as well as for snacks in between. To flush toxins, drink half of your body weight in ounces of water, in addition to the juices you consume. A sample daily plan follows.

Your Fast-Day Juicing Schedule

Wake Up
12–16 ounces warm water with the juice of ½ lemon

Breakfast
12–16 ounces fresh vegetable + fruit juice

1 Hour Later (8-9 a.m.)
12–16 ounces water (Sip over the course of the hour.)

Midmorning
12–16 ounces fresh vegetable + fruit juice

Late Morning (10-11 a.m.)
12–16 ounces water or herbal tea (Sip over the course of the hour.)

Lunch
12–16 ounces fresh vegetable + fruit juice

1 Hour Later (1-2 p.m.)
12–16 ounces water (Sip over the course of the hour.)

Midafternoon
12–16 ounces vegetable + fruit juice

Late Afternoon (4-5 p.m.)
12–16 ounces water or herbal tea (Sip over the course of the hour.)

Dinner
12–16 ounces vegetable + fruit juice

1 Hour Later (6-7 p.m.)
12–16 ounces water or herbal tea

Note: It's important to drink your juice all at one time, as if it were your meal, so that your pancreas won't be pumping out insulin all day long.

(continued on page 152)

Seven Simple Vegetable and Fruit Juice Recipes

Give these basic recipes a try, and feel free to experiment. The more fruit you add, the sweeter the juice will be. The less fruit, the less fructose you'll consume. As always, the key is to find the right balance, where the juice tastes delicious and you're not overloading your body with fruit sugars. Find combinations that suit your taste buds and make you feel energized. When you fast, it's best to use all organic ingredients. If you can't find them at your local grocery store or farmers' market, peel the apples and pears, and forgo the strawberries and spinach. (Both of these are sprayed heavily.)

Fruity Green Power

3 leaves organic chard

1/2 bunch organic cilantro

1 crispy organic pear, seeds removed

4 organic strawberries

1" organic ginger

Freshener

5 leaves organic romaine lettuce

1/2 bunch organic spinach

1/2 bunch organic watercress

1 organic carrot

2 crispy organic apples, seeds removed

Bok Joy

3 leaves organic beet greens

3 leaves organic bok choy

1/2 organic cucumber

1 organic apple, seeds removed

1 carrot

Spicy Kale

2 leaves organic kale

1/2 bunch organic spinach

1 organic apple, seeds removed

1 organic carrot

1" organic ginger

Pinch of cayenne (optional)

Green Pom Cooler

1 bunch organic spinach

$\frac{1}{3}$ small bunch of organic cilantro

3 leaves organic kale

2 organic carrots

1 organic cucumber

1 organic orange, seeds removed

Seeds from 1 pomegranate

Apple Power

4 leaves organic kale

$\frac{1}{4}$ head organic cabbage

$\frac{1}{2}$ organic cucumber

3 organic apples, seeds removed

1 organic orange, seeds removed

$\frac{1}{2}$ organic lemon, seeds removed

Green Pom Seed

4 leaves organic kale

4 leaves organic bok choy

1 organic carrot

Seeds from 2 pomegranates

There are limitless combinations, so have fun creating your own recipes. You'll quickly discover which combinations you prefer. Some tips for choosing ingredients:

- Ginger and lemon can be added to stimulate cleansing.
- Ginger aids in circulation, warming your body and flushing out toxins.
- Lemons help to dislodge and eliminate mucus and fat, cleansing your colon and strengthening your liver.

Fasting Option #2:
The Master Cleanse Lemonade

The Master Cleanse was developed as a stomach ulcer cure in 1940 by Stanley Burroughs, an early advocate of natural health who believed in the body's natural ability to heal itself. In 1976, he published his fasting diet in *The Master Cleanser*[24] and promoted it not only for ulcers but also for weight loss and degenerative diseases. Since then, thousands have used the Master Cleanse as a fasting technique. For example, Dr. Elson Haas has written much about this in his books, and he has done the cleanse every year since 1975.

The Master Cleanse fast consists of drinking eight to twelve 8-ounce glasses of a spicy homemade lemonade over the course of the day. Between lemonade drinks, consume half your body weight in ounces of purified water. (So if you weigh 140 pounds, drink at least 70 ounces of water, in addition to your 2½ to 3 quarts of lemonade.)

To make 1 serving of the Master Cleanse Lemonade, combine the following:

- 2 tablespoons freshly squeezed lemon juice. Use fresh lemons, preferably organic, not bottled juice. Limes may be substituted. Lemon zest and pulp may be added.

- 1–2 tablespoons pure Grade B maple syrup, which has more color and nutrients than Grade A. (But if you already have Grade A syrup in your fridge, you may use it.)

- A pinch of cayenne pepper. You can begin with a smaller amount if the taste and spiciness aren't to your liking.

- 10–12 ounces of medium-warm, hot, or room temperature spring water.

In *The Detox Diet*, Elson Haas, MD, offers this suggestion when drinking the lemonade: Rinse your mouth with water after each glass to prevent the lemon juice from hurting the enamel of your teeth.

The Science Behind the Master Cleanse Fast

The Master Cleanse lemonade is so effective because its ingredients promote cleansing and healing while stimulating your digestive system. Here's a look at how each ingredient contributes to your health.

Cayenne Pepper. As we've learned, cayenne pepper has two special properties: its healing properties and its heat. Capsaicin is the phytochemical in chile peppers that makes them spicy and provides heat. It's the heat in cayenne that helps boost metabolism and regulate blood sugar levels.[25] It also has diuretic effects, so it helps clear excess water.

A study at Manchester Metropolitan University in England showed that capsaicin not only increases your body's metabolism but also triggers your body to burn lipids (body fat) and reduce appetite. Researchers showed that calorie-burning capsaicin, one of nature's stimulants, works by causing an adrenaline release similar to your body's fight-or-flight mechanism, which increases energy production and reduces appetite.

Make a Big Batch}

If you'd like to make a full day's supply of your fasting lemonade, combine the first three ingredients into a concentrate of lemon juice, maple syrup, and cayenne. Measure your water (2 to 2 1/2 quarts) in a pitcher to make sure you drink the entire amount over the course of the day. Wait to add your water to each serving, because cayenne's heat becomes more intense in water. Mix 3 tablespoons of the concentrate with 10 to 12 ounces of water just before drinking. Your ingredients and water can sit out on the counter during the day.

A Full Batch of Concentrate for the Day

1 cup freshly squeezed lemon juice

1/2 cup maple syrup

1 1/2 teaspoon cayenne pepper (go slowly, adding only as much as you can tolerate)

Plus, capsaicin affects your body's hormone levels, further reducing appetite. And in a 2009 study of 27 healthy volunteers at Hokkaido University Graduate School of Medicine in Sapporo, Japan, researchers found that consuming a combination of capsaicin and green tea led subjects to feel less hungry and consume fewer calories. Finally, a 2009 Danish study found that capsaicin may help decrease ghrelin, the hormone involved in promoting hunger.[26]

Fresh Lemon. Here are just a few of the many benefits lemon juice provides: First, lemons are high in the antioxidant vitamin C, which provides anti-inflammatory properties, strengthening your immune function. Lemons also contain saponins—antimicrobial compounds that may offer protection from colds and flu.[27]

Even though lemons are so tart, they're quite alkalizing. With both citric and ascorbic acid, they're quickly metabolized, so their mineral content can alkalize your blood. Because lemons are internal cleansers for your GI tract, bloodstream, kidneys, and liver, they induce internal cleansing on a cellular level to detox your organs.

Another plus for lemons: They aid in digestion. That's because of the citrus flavonoids, citric and ascorbic acid, that they contain. Lemon juice enhances the production of hydrochloric acid in your stomach, which helps your digestion.

Maple Syrup. Maple syrup provides calories, sweetness, and antioxidants—it has as many antioxidants as broccoli or tomatoes! The darker the grade of syrup, the higher the antioxidant activity. As a natural sweetener, flavorful maple syrup is lower in calories than honey.

Your Fast Day Lemonade Schedule

Drink as much lemonade as you like each day, aiming for at least 2½ quarts, drinking between 12 and 16 ounces every other hour. In addition, drink at least equal amounts of water. You'll be drinking some liquid every hour. Your total liquid intake over the course of the day will be 84 to 112 ounces water and 72 to 96 ounces Master Cleanse Lemonade.

Wake Up
12–16 ounces water

Breakfast (7–8 a.m.)
12–16 ounces Master Cleanse Lemonade

1 Hour Later (8–9 a.m.)
12–16 ounces water (Sip over the course of the hour.)

Midmorning (9–10 a.m.)
12–16 ounces Master Cleanse Lemonade

Late Morning (10–11 a.m.)
12–16 ounces water or herbal tea (Sip over the course of the hour.)

Lunch (12–1 p.m.)
12–16 ounces Master Cleanse Lemonade

1 Hour Later (1–2 p.m.)
12–16 ounces water

Midafternoon (2–3 p.m.)
12–16 ounces Master Cleanse Lemonade

Late Afternoon (3–4 p.m.)
12–16 ounces water or herbal tea (Sip over the course of the hour.)

Dinner (5–6 p.m.)
12–16 ounces Master Cleanse Lemonade

1 Hour Later (6–7 p.m.)
12–16 ounces water or herbal tea

Snack (7–8 p.m.)
12–16 ounces Master Cleanse Lemonade

Before Bedtime (8–9 p.m.)
12–16 ounces water

Option #3: LiverUp! Pomegranate Punch Fast

Here's how to mix up a batch of the LiverUp! Pomegranate Punch:

8 ounces unsweetened pomegranate juice

2 quarts spring water

1 teaspoon fresh ginger, very finely chopped

1/2 teaspoon organic ground cinnamon

1 teaspoon organic whole cloves

1/4 cup freshly squeezed lemon juice

4–6 tablespoons ground flax or chia seeds

Stevia to taste (liquid tincture is best, but packets are fine)

In a small saucepan, bring the juice and water to a boil. Reduce heat to low.

If you have a tea ball or piece of cheesecloth, place the ginger, cinnamon, and cloves inside it and add it to the pan. If not, you can put the spices directly into the water. Let simmer for 5 to 10 minutes. Let cool to room temperature and strain or remove the spices. Stir in the lemon juice and seeds and add stevia to taste. Pomegranate punch doesn't need refrigeration.

The Science behind the LiverUp! Pomegranate Fast

Pomegranate juice is a recent star in the nutrition galaxy. It provides some of the highest levels of antioxidants, beating out green tea, red wine, and cranberry juice.[28] Pomegranate's antioxidants thin your blood by inhibiting both excessive blood cell clotting and LDL oxidation, thus helping to prevent cardiovascular disease. LDL (bad) cholesterol is only damaging in the body when it's oxidized, so pomegranate juice, which prevents LDL oxidation, is beneficial for cardiovascular health.[29] Pomegranate juice contains vitamins A, C, and E, which act as antioxidants, scavenging free radicals that can cause cellular damage.

An Israeli study has shown that the sugars in pomegranate juice not only maintain low glucose levels but also lower blood pressure and protect against atherosclerosis—a hardening of the arteries caused by continually high glucose levels. Both hypertension and atherosclerosis lead to heart disease and stroke. This condition happens when sugars are not only high but also present in harmful forms. The sugars in pomegranate juice, the study found, are attached to unique antioxidants that protect against plaque buildup in your arteries and veins.[30] Pomegranate juice is an excellent fruit juice for fasting. Its antioxidants protect your body against free radicals, and its sugars maintain fluid and flexible arteries without raising glucose levels.

Fresh Ginger. Ginger is warming and healing to your digestive tract, possessing many anti-inflammatory, antiviral, and antimicrobial properties.[31] Like pomegranate juice, ginger supports detoxification by nourishing your liver and supporting circulation. The root has been shown to inhibit the oxidation of LDL, potentially reduce levels of triglycerides, improve carbohydrate and lipid metabolism, and slow the development of atherosclerosis, heart disease, diabetes, and nonalcoholic fatty liver disease.[32]

In a study published in the *Indian Journal of Pharmaceutical Sciences,* ginger was tested on animals with liver disease. A daily dose of 250 milligrams significantly reversed liver damage and moved blood composition toward normal.[33] In addition, ginger has been shown to support your liver's ability to detox your body. Research at Cairo University in Egypt showed that ginger extract increased levels of antioxidant enzymes, including glutathione peroxidase, which is essential for a high-functioning liver.[34]

Cinnamon. Cinnamon boosts your metabolism and helps lower blood sugar. In addition, it may also help your body utilize fat.[35]

Cloves. Cloves are powerful antioxidants and are an excellent source of manganese, a trace element that regulates the digestive system, aiding in the absorption of fat during the process of digestion, reducing constipation and bowel discomfort. Manganese also helps your body digest food more efficiently. According to researchers at Oregon State University, manganese-activated enzymes aid in cholesterol, amino acid, glutamine, and carbohydrate metabolism. One particular enzyme, superoxide dismutase (MnSOD) is worth noting. This enzyme is essential for healthy functioning of the brain and used to treat nervous system disorders. MnSOD is the primary antioxidant enzyme that protects cells from oxidative stress, scavenging free radicals throughout the body, including the neural pathways. Remember that oxidation by-products like free radicals are everywhere in your body, and your brain can be negatively affected just as easily as other parts of your body, so powerful antioxidants like MnSOD come to the rescue. Aside from its antioxidant role, manganese can also bind with neurotransmitters and speed up cognitive function.[36]

Plus, manganese supports liver function, playing a critical role in the metabolism of glutamine, the most abundant amino acid in your body.[37] It also aids in regulating glucose metabolism, providing critical energy throughout your body. When your body absorbs and utilizes glucose properly, there is less buildup, which helps you maintain balanced blood sugar levels.[38]

Cloves have antiseptic, germicidal, and anti-inflammatory properties that help fight infections, relieve digestive problems, and lower systemic inflammation; their antiviral and cleansing properties purify your body and augment your resistance to disease. And cloves are hugely beneficial during fasting because they help purify blood, stabilize blood sugar levels, stimulate your circulatory system, clear your mind, reduce fatigue, and encourage your digestive system to eliminate food and toxins.

Ground Flax or Chia Seeds. Flax and chia seeds both provide omega-3 essential fatty acids and soluble and insoluble fiber, as well as

{Supplements and Medications

Supplements are not recommended during your 1- or 2-day fast. On an empty stomach, supplements can stress your digestive system and may cause nausea. You can begin taking them again once you return to your cleansing foods, but skip them during your fast. If you're on prescription drugs, consult your physician before fasting. It's critical to obtain sound advice about these medications.

lignans, those estrogen-regulating substances that have antiviral, antibacterial, and antifungal properties.[39]

Stevia. Stevia is a plant-based sweetener that balances blood sugar and restores insulin sensitivity. Unlike other sweeteners, stevia hasn't been implicated in any cancers.[40]

Your Fast Day Pomegranate Punch Schedule

Alternate drinking water with Pomegranate Punch every other hour, taking in some liquid every hour. Your total daily liquid intake will be 84 to 112 ounces of water and 72 to 96 ounces of Pomegranate Punch. Make up the whole batch at the beginning of the day and drink a serving every other hour.

Wake Up
16–20 ounces water.

Breakfast (7–8 a.m.)
12–16 ounces Pomegranate Punch

1 Hour Later (8–9 a.m.)
16–20 ounces water (Sip over the course of the hour.)

Midmorning (9–10 a.m.)
12–16 ounces Pomegranate Punch

Late Morning (10–11 a.m.)
16–20 ounces water or herbal tea (Sip over the course of the hour.)

Lunch (12–1 p.m.)
12–16 ounces Pomegranate Punch

1 Hour Later (1–2 p.m.)
16–20 ounces water

Midafternoon (2–3 p.m.)
12–16 ounces Pomegranate Punch

Late Afternoon (3–4 p.m.)
12–16 ounces water/herbal tea (Sip over the course of the hour.)

Dinner (5-6 p.m.)
12–16 ounces Pomegranate Punch

1 Hour Later (6-7 p.m.)
12–16 ounces water or herbal tea

Snack (7-8 p.m.)
12–16 ounces Pomegranate Punch

Before Bedtime (8-9 p.m.)
12–16 ounces water

Fasting: A Journey of Discovery

Choose the healing option that "feels" best to you—usually you can rely on your intuition about what's right. Through experimentation, intention, and awareness, you'll discover your individual nutritional needs and meet them with ease.

Having a set plan for the day can be very helpful. Observe, listen to, and honor your body. This day is an opportunity to reconnect with yourself and your true nature.

Fasting can become an effective practice to incorporate into your life, helping you pause and allowing your body's systems to rest, restore, and rejuvenate.

Remember: You're taking this day or two to honor yourself in body, mind, and spirit. Walk through it mindfully, intentionally, and purposefully. In the next chapter, we'll look at ways to nourish yourself during this very important time.

The LiverUp! Diaries

ANDY MCCORMACK, 55

Dynamic Duo

Lost: 12 pounds

Heart health: Positive changes toward improvement

Energy: Increased

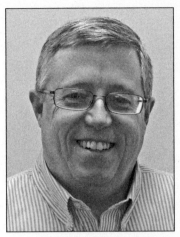

I did the cleanse because I just wanted to feel better—and I did. I was on medication for high blood pressure, and though I didn't monitor my numbers before and after the cleanse, the numbers I did pay attention to were on the scale. Over the course of the cleanse, I lost 12 pounds, and I know that's a step in the right direction for my heart health. I even noticed that my pants were looser, and I just felt better all around.

It was an interesting experience, and at first it was a little daunting, but it was fun to do it as a team with my wife. We'd go shopping at Whole Foods Market and try vegetables we'd never tried before, like kale. It was kind of an adventure. We really embraced the smoothie recipe and got into the whey protein and all of the fruits—that's something we've carried on from the cleanse. We still crank out smoothies almost every morning for breakfast.

The cleanse really opened our eyes to a lot of things—it was fascinating to learn what foods do for our organs, especially our livers. We really took it to heart—it helped to know exactly why you don't want to eat a block of cheese with a beer every night. Cutting out cheese and alcohol was a challenge, but other things were easy. I don't drink coffee, so I didn't have to suffer from caffeine withdrawal like other people do.

My wife and I even did the fast day, and we got through it pretty well! When the cleanse was all over, I had a lot more energy. I haven't stuck to everything on the eating plan, but I have picked up some healthier habits and I really think that the small changes have made a difference in my life. Today, I'm much more aware of what I'm eating and what it takes to live a healthy life.

CHAPTER 7

Cleansing Your Heart, Mind, and Soul:
Emotional, Mental, and Spiritual Detoxing

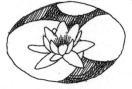

In addition to detoxifying your organs, tissues, and cells, cleansing helps you to reconnect with both your natural rhythm and the rhythm of the earth. The process of nourishing your body with special cleansing, healing, and strengthening foods allows you the space and time to return to your center and step back from some of the influences of our toxic world.

For author and holistic physician Gabriel Cousens, MD, who helps his patients weave together their physical, emotional, mental, and spiritual health, cleansing and fasting are essential practices for living a healthy life.

> . . . Fasting, in a larger context, means to abstain from that which is toxic to mind, body, and soul . . . [eliminating] physical, emotional, and mental toxins from our organism, rather than simply cutting down on or stopping food intake. Fasting for spiritual purposes . . . can be a great revival to those of us who have been putting our energy outward.[1]

Detoxing offers the opportunity to slow down and to see your path more clearly. It challenges you to connect with your inner strength as

163

you forgo old habits and learn to live with renewed energy and clarity. To support you during your cleanse and beyond, this chapter offers pathways to a healthier life by balancing your emotions, calming your mind, and renewing your spirit.

Overcoming Emotional, Spiritual, and Mental Blocks

As the Dalai Lama says, "We can never obtain peace in the outer world until we make peace within ourselves."[2] To do that, though, it's important to identify the obstacles to peace. Let's take a look at some of the big ones.

We Suppress Our Emotions

Sometimes our emotions can seem toxic and uncomfortable, so we avoid experiencing them by denying or suppressing them. Research confirms that unresolved issues and emotional baggage affect all aspects of our lives and can result in a variety of serious symptoms. And the reverse is also true: Your gut contains neurotransmitters that affect your emotional well-being, so it's easy to see how these aspects of your life are so closely intertwined.

Not only does your gut contain much of your body's immune system, it also contains cells that carry emotions to your brain. As a mass, these cells form an aggregate of neural tissue, filled with important neurotransmitters that convey feelings and emotions to your brain. This network of neurons lining your gut is so extensive that it's known as the "second brain."[3]

Your second brain, or enteric nervous system, consists of sheaths of neurons embedded in the walls of the long tube of your gut—your entire digestive system, or alimentary canal—measuring about 9 meters end to end, from esophagus to anus. It contains some 100 million neurons, more than are found in your spinal cord or peripheral nervous system, enabling you to "feel" the inner world of your gut and significantly affecting your emotions. Ever experience the flutter of butterflies in your stomach before a stressful event? That's one example of your enteric nervous system at work. Your emotional health may rely on messages relayed from your brain below to your brain above.[4] The relationship between these two brains—in your head and in your gut—has been linked with both mental health issues, such as anxiety and depression, and physical health issues, like irritable bowel syndrome (IBS), ulcers, and Parkinson's disease.[5]

Another factor affecting this relationship between emotional stress and physical distress is the neurotransmitter serotonin. A whopping 95 percent of this chemical, which is responsible for feelings of happiness and contentment, lives in the gut. The digestive process begins when a specialized cell emits serotonin into the wall of your gut. It's like a messenger, keeping the brain in your skull informed about what's happening in your "second" brain below.[6]

Your emotions, which are directly influenced by your two brains, manifest themselves in your physical body. And if you don't allow yourself to really feel your feelings, they never leave you, resulting in self-sabotaging behavior that can lead to addiction and illness.[7]

Though we often recoil in fear when toxic feelings rise, when we fully experience our feelings, we can free ourselves from their destructive grip. Cleansing offers an opportunity to work through your emotions with clarity and a peaceful heart. When you nurture your body with healing and cleansing foods, you learn how food can nourish and sustain you rather than sabotage or punish you. You begin to realize that your relationship with food can teach you about your relationship with life.

We Deceive Our Mind

When confronted with a challenge, your mind steps up to the task of solving, organizing, and planning. But your mind doesn't serve you well when it locks into negative thought patterns, opinions, and judgments.

Jon Kabat-Zinn, a molecular biologist who teaches mindfulness meditation as a technique to help people cope with stress, pain, and illness, contends that we live in a dream reality, unable and unwilling to see through the vapor, due to our attachment to the dream.[8] When we're living in a dreamlike state, we're not fully aware, nor present in the moment, because we're too busy denying reality or pushing it away.

Mindfulness, on the other hand, is being fully awake, noticing and being present in the moment at hand. For Kabat-Zinn, practicing mindfulness means "giving up coercing, resisting, or struggling, in exchange for something more powerful and wholesome which comes out of allowing things to be as they are without getting caught up in your attraction to or rejection of them, in the intrinsic stickiness of wanting, of liking and disliking."[9]

And what and how you eat impacts your ability to be present to yourself and to the moment. When you cleanse your liver—and thus your body—the fog clears from your mind, making it more lucid and allowing you to think more clearly and perceive yourself more honestly. In a study at the David Geffen School of Medicine at UCLA, researchers analyzed more than 160 studies about food's effect on the brain. The studies indicate that a whole foods diet, rich in omega-3 fatty acids, antioxidants, and polyphenols, strengthens the connections between the synapses, enhancing cognitive abilities, protecting your brain from damage, and counteracting the effects of aging.

Researchers confirmed that diets high in trans fats and saturated fats adversely affect your brain's synapses, which impairs your ability to think clearly. Your brain, in particular, is sensitive to oxidative damage caused by free radical formation, while foods high in antioxidants (such as berries, beans, broccoli, and Brussels sprouts) benefit your brain. Another important finding: Consuming too many calories can make your synapses less flexible, and that makes your cells more vulnerable to free radical damage. But just cutting down calories a little bit seems to protect your brain.[10] The bottom line: When your brain is functioning well, you can be awake and present—to yourself, and to life as it is in the moment.

We Ignore the Spirit

Our spirit is as close to us as our breath. In fact, many ancient religions define spirit as breath, linking both to life itself. Yet many of us ignore our spirit, hold our breath, and walk through our lives in a semiconscious dreamland.

But what we think and feel has a profound effect on our physical and spiritual health. The Buddhist tradition teaches that we create much of our own suffering by not accepting the present moment. In *Peace Is Every Breath*, Buddhist monk Thich Nhat Hanh writes:

> All of us need to have a spiritual dimension in our lives. We need spiritual practice. If that practice is regular and solid, we will be able to transform the fear, anger, and despair in us and overcome the difficulties we all encounter in daily life.[11]

For Thich Nhat Hanh, the spiritual journey is about waking up and becoming present to the moment, to ourselves, and to one another. Mindfulness and concentration, he insists, are integral to our spiritual practice, so whatever we do, we must choose to do it with mindfulness and focus, transforming our actions into a spiritual practice. Breathing mindfully, walking mindfully, driving mindfully—all become our spiritual practice, promising to bring more "serenity, acceptance, and joy into our lives."[12]

Cleansing encourages you to be intentional and conscious about what, when, and how you're eating. In turn, this intentionality increases your moment-to-moment awareness, enabling you to breathe in a sense of calm and creating a reservoir of peace and serenity for your mind and spirit.

We Numb Ourselves with Food

Racing through our lives, we seem to worry that if we were to slow down, our house of cards would fall. So we stay busy, work harder and longer, and don't even take time out for a quiet meal. Often, we even numb ourselves with food. Here's how.

Processed foods—the flour and sweets many of us consume lots of—turn to sugar in our blood. In addition to triggering an insulin release, sugar increases two chemicals that affect our sense of well-being—serotonin and beta-endorphins. When these chemical levels are high, we experience a "sugar high" that makes us feel confident and calm. But each of these two chemicals anesthetizes our brains and thus our emotions in different ways.

Serotonin. Remember that 95 percent of your body's serotonin is housed in your gut. As a neurotransmitter, it facilitates communication between nerve cells and muscles. Often called the "feel good" chemical, when it's at an ideal level, you feel relaxed and hopeful, creative, thoughtful, positive, and focused, and you have strong control over your impulses.

But when your serotonin levels are low, you become more impulsive because insufficient serotonin levels impede you from making sound choices. According to Mayo Clinic nutritionists Jennifer Nelson, MS, RD, and Katherine Zeratsky, RD, you may feel depressed and find yourself craving bread, pasta, candy, or processed foods, since your brain knows that the refined carbs in these foods will temporarily raise your serotonin levels.[13]

Your body manufactures serotonin from the amino acid tryptophan, derived from dietary protein you consume. But that tryptophan doesn't automatically travel to your brain because of the blood-brain barrier, which filters out potentially harmful substances.

When you consume carbohydrates—especially refined carbs like cookies and pasta—your blood sugar rises, signaling your pancreas to secrete insulin. As insulin goes to work, it lowers these sugar levels in your bloodstream and reduces the levels of many amino acids, including glutamine and alanine. Because tryptophan competes with other amino acids to pass through the blood-brain barrier, fewer amino acids to compete with means that tryptophan can now enter your brain, increasing the amount of serotonin. So sugar and refined carbs pave a direct path for tryptophan to travel to your brain, increase serotonin, and make you feel better. That's the chemistry behind the sugar high.

Beta-Endorphins. Beta-endorphins are the brain chemicals that act as natural painkillers. They affect your self-esteem, confidence, and sense of connection and are responsible for the euphoria, or runner's high, you feel after a challenging workout. Sugar, along with chocolate, alcohol, and even heroin, creates a flood of beta-endorphins, numbing emotional pain and providing a sense of comfort.

As sugar creates more serotonin and beta-endorphins in your brain, you may crave it and use it like a drug. You love the "sugar buzz" that makes you feel happy, or even a little high. Or you may experience a sense of calm, focus, and clarity—for about 30 minutes. Then your blood sugar and brain chemical levels drop and you experience a sugar crash that makes you feel fatigued, irritable, and unfocused. And you'll do anything for another bag of chips, piece of cake, or giant cup of soda.

The cycle will continue unless you commit to eliminating sugar and refined foods for a time. When you do, you will experience not only a physical detox, but an emotional, mental, and spiritual detox, as well. The LiverUp! Cleanse offers a path that detoxes all these aspects of your life.

Cleanse the Body, Quiet the Mind

Your hectic life and your mindless eating disconnects you from yourself, keeping your inner life at bay. When you rush through your days and munch in front of the TV, you're not fully enjoying the amazing experience of living.

Cleansing, though, forces you to slow down and practice awareness and mindfulness. To consume an array of healthy foods, you have to practice complete awareness and intentionality throughout the day, rather than cruising through the kitchen or drive-thru for a bag of chips or an order of fries. Instead, you have to plan your next meal, your next snack, even your next glass of water. This intentionality requires you to slow down—and the act of slowing down is a gift to your soul. For 12 days, cleansing allows you to put aside your busyness and breathe. If you've ever had a massage, you know that it not only releases tension from your muscles, but it also allows for emotional and spiritual release. Cleansing your body is similar. As your tissues release chemicals, toxins, and fat, emotions and thoughts buried deep in the same tissues tend to rise to the surface. With a clearer mind, you can work to end destructive behavior.

Techniques to Calm and Nurture

The LiverUp! Cleanse offers practices to support you emotionally, mentally, and spiritually during your 12 days of cleansing. See which ones resonate with you. Take what you need and leave the rest.

Observe and Record Your Emotions and Thoughts

Even if you don't think of yourself as a writer, try recording in a journal—or in a daily letter to yourself—what you feel and experience as you move through these days of renewal. You may even want to express your experience through art, perhaps as a series of sketches, a collage, or even a scrapbook. Or use the journal pages that begin on page 312 of this book.

Let your emotions and thoughts flow through your heart and mind and right onto the paper. These writings are just for you, so they don't have to make sense to anyone else. Whatever your feelings, allow them to spring forth.

Begin Each Day with Mindful, Conscious Breathing

In yoga, this breathing practice is called pranayama, which is a combination of three Sanskrit words.

Prana: life force or life energy

Yama: discipline or control

Ayama: expansion, nonrestraint, or extension

By using pranayama, you can extend your life force—the vital energy force that circulates throughout your body and through all living things—by controlling your breath.

Breathing is one of the few autonomic functions of the body that you can actually control. In addition to its physiological benefits, intentional, controlled breathing reduces stress and quiets the mind, allowing you to feel a sense of calm and serenity. In a randomized controlled trial, researchers showed that 8 weeks of relaxation training, including instruction on breathing techniques, significantly reduced systolic blood pressure in individuals with systolic hypertension, enabling almost a third of them to eliminate one or more of their antihypertensive medications.[14]

When you encounter stress, your sympathetic nervous system (SNS) takes over, and one of your first responses is to hold your breath or take rapid, shallow breaths while your mind races to predict what's likely to happen. Your SNS is what's behind your fight-or-flight response, which signals your adrenal glands to pump cortisol and adrenaline into your system. Adrenaline's task is to speed up your heart rate, elevate your blood pressure, and boost your energy. Cortisol is your stress hormone; it provides an immediate surge of energy, while minimizing the effects of insulin. When this fight-or-flight scenario goes on for a long time—or happens frequently—it can lead to some serious health problems. That's because when blood sugars stay high, your pancreas secretes more and more insulin to cells that have become insulin resistant. And that can bring about weight gain or, eventually, diabetes. Plus, prolonged stress can also burden your immune system, and that can make you catch lots of different illnesses. Your body's natural response to danger is a good thing. The challenge is that many of us live under constant stress, which triggers an ongoing release of both cortisol and adrenaline.

Under normal circumstances, your body's stress-response system is usually short-term: The danger passes and your hormones quietly get back to normal. As adrenaline and cortisol levels drop, your heart rate and blood pressure return to normal, communicating to your body that it's safe for all its systems to resume their regular functions. But when stressors are constantly present, that fight-or-flight response is continuously triggered. When your stress-response system is on constant alert, your body gets flooded with cortisol and other stress hormones, which can disrupt almost all of your body's processes. And this ongoing output of stress hormones puts you at increased risk of numerous health problems, including anxiety, depression, digestive problems, heart disease, sleep problems, weight gain, and memory and concentration impairment.

But deep, mindful, abdominal breathing, says Mark Liponis, MD, author of *UltraLongevity,* activates the vagus nerve, kick-starting your parasympathetic nervous system (PNS) and prompting the relaxation response, which is the opposite of your stress response. Conscious breathing rebalances your body chemistry by supplying your brain with ample oxygen and allowing your PNS to take over, taking you from a state of high alert to a calm state, where you can react rationally.[15]

In 1921, German physiologist Otto Loewi first discovered a link between the vagus nerve and heart rate reduction. The vagus nerve extends from the brain stem down to all your internal organs. It carries information from your nervous system to your brain and from your brain down to your gut. Specifically, Loewi and his team determined that when the vagus nerve was stimulated, it triggered the release of a chemical they called "vaggusstuff." That chemical was later identified by scientists as acetylcholine, the first neurotransmitter.[16] Otto's research won him the Nobel Prize in 1936. A more recent study at the Feinstein Institute for Medical Research in Manhasset, New York, has found that acetylcholine has relaxing and calming qualities, which you can activate by deep breaths and long exhalations. Plus, acetylcholine reduces inflammation, which, as we've learned, can be triggered by stress.[17]

Research has also linked the vagus nerve to improved neurogenesis, increased brain-derived neurotrophic factor output (BDNF is like super-fertilizer for your brain cells), and repair of brain tissue, as well as to actual regeneration throughout the body. For example, scientists have found that stem cells are directly connected to the vagus nerve, and activating the vagus nerve can also stimulate stem cells to produce new cells to repair and rebuild your organs.[18]

Neuroscience confirms that you can transform your internal responses to the external events you can't control. Before-and-after brain scans show that an ongoing practice of mindfulness and meditation changes your brain chemistry and activates your left prefrontal lobe, the brain's "happiness center." There's a growing body of research on the benefits of mindfulness and the ability of the practice to shift the brain.

Researchers at Massachusetts General Hospital, for example, studied 26 overstressed but otherwise healthy businesspeople. After 8 weeks of mindfulness meditation training, participants experienced an increased ability to manage difficult emotions and greater emotional stability and sense of self. They spent an average of 27 minutes daily practicing mindfulness exercises. At the end of 2 months, their responses to a mindfulness questionnaire indicated significant improvements compared with pre-participation responses.[19]

If you engage in the spiritual practice of mindful breathing and meditation, you can shift the way your brain functions. For example: Studies conducted at the National Institutes of Health suggest that mindfulness practices may help people manage stress, cope better with serious illness, and reduce anxiety and depression. One NIH-supported study found a link between mindfulness meditation and measurable changes in brain regions involved in memory, learning, and emotion.[20] And another study reported that mindfulness practices may reduce anxiety and hostility among urban youth and lead to reduced stress, fewer fights, and better relationships.[21]

To truly experience the benefits of mindfulness, though, consistency is key. You wouldn't expect to see much benefit if you got on your yoga mat only once a week, and the same is true with mindfulness training. You should practice and cultivate it daily, choosing in every moment to bring your attention to the present. When you do this, you're actively involved in shifting your mind and brain to foster peace and inner ease.

Mindfulness Meditations

As the sutras say, "Now is the time." So let's start now. Here are some breathing practices for you to try. To figure out which one is best for you, practice one of these exercises each day for a week and observe how each one affects your body, breath, and mind. You can do them at just about any time of day, though avoid practicing immediately after a large meal.

Breathing Exercise #1: Belly (or Diaphragmatic) Breathing

Pranayama begins with observation. Relax your entire body and observe your breath. Don't try to control your breath—simply notice it. Notice where your breath resides in your body: Does it land in your lungs or travel down to your belly?

Now, place one hand on your abdomen and close your eyes. Take a deep breath in through your nose. Take the breath into your lungs, fill your lungs, and then take that same breath deeper, down into your belly. Expand your belly with this inhalation. Can you feel the expansion? If not, imagine a balloon inflating in your belly when you breathe in.

Now exhale, and as you let your breath out, feel your belly flatten, as your balloon deflates. Again, inhale through your nose and expand your belly with your breath, filling your balloon. Exhale, deflating your balloon.

Try to make your exhalation the same length as your inhalation. Gradually begin to make your breathing as relaxed and smooth as possible, introducing a slight pause after each in-breath and out-breath.

Take 10 breath cycles. Notice the quality of your breath. What is the rhythm of your inhalation and exhalation? What is the texture of your breath: Is it long and smooth, or is it a bit short and rough? Just observe.

If you notice any tension in your body, or find yourself short of breath, just relax and stop for a while. Aim to keep your breath calm and fluid.

When your breath is relaxed and you feel calm and comfortable, you'll become more aware of your body's movements—your belly expands as you inhale and contracts as you exhale. Gently, try to further expand your belly as you inhale and contract it even more as you exhale to stimulate your vagus nerve. That signals your parasympathetic nervous system to take over, generating a sense of calm and ease. Continue for 10 more deep breath cycles.

For a fast mini-relaxation break any time, take a deep breath and release it slowly—like a letting-go breath. Try counting backward from 10 to 1, with one number on each out-breath. By the time you get to 1, you'll notice that your breath is slower and more regular and that your body and mind are relaxing. With practice, you'll form the habit of breathing from your diaphragm most of the time, which keeps you from taking shallow breaths from the top of your lungs, depriving your body of essential oxygen.

Breathing Exercise #2: Mindful Breathing

Mindful breathing offers a calm, nonjudging awareness, allowing thoughts and feelings to come and go without dwelling on them.

To begin, sit comfortably on a cushion or in a chair, with your spine and neck straight, lifting up from your pelvis. Roll your shoulders down your back and relax them. Bring your chin to parallel with the floor and tuck it slightly in, toward your chest.

Set a timer. Begin with 5, 10, or 20 minutes—whatever feels most reasonable. Commit to this time and let the timer indicate when your sitting is complete.

Close your eyes and begin the exercise by noticing the sounds in and outside of the room. Let your mind be open and sensitive to what's happening around you.

Now bring your attention to your breathing. Notice the movement of your breath in your body. Be aware of your breath's movement as physical sensations in your belly. If you're unable to sense the movement in your belly, notice instead the way your chest moves. Let your breath flow naturally and rhythmically in and down into your pelvis, then up to your chest and out your nose. Simply notice it, without judging it.

Next, notice the texture of your breath. It may be short or long, shallow or deep, tense or even, strained or easy. Acknowledge it as it is and let it be. Stay attuned to your breath and allow it to keep you present to the moment.

Now take your attention to your body, noticing any tightness or tension. Allow yourself to physically relax, and acknowledge these sensations as you encounter them. Don't struggle with anything. When feelings arise and your thoughts take you out of your body, bring your awareness back to your breath. Notice your emotions and feelings, then bring your attention back to your breathing, as if you're on the outside looking in.

Thoughts will come into your mind, but simply notice them. If your mind wanders off into the future or back into the past, note it as "thinking," "planning," or "remembering." The mind is programmed to do these things. Let go of your judgment and simply notice, bringing your attention back to your breath and to the present moment.

Allow your thoughts to come and go. They will rise naturally to the surface and pass. Simply allow the thoughts to be present, notice them, and allow them to float past, and turn your attention back to your breath.

Thoughts will come and go. They will enter your awareness and your mind will catch them. Each time you notice your attention is elsewhere, bring it gently back to your breath. Allow your breath to be your anchor. Let the movement of your breath in your belly or chest be your main focus. When you catch yourself traveling into your thoughts, let it be an opportunity to wake up and return to center.

Let your attention be consistent from moment to moment. Try to experience each inhalation and each exhalation with an open heart and mind. As you meet and greet the experience of your breath in an open and accepting way, your breath and your experience become one. There is only now, this breath, and this experience. Be whole with your breath, breathing with an open, focused mind.

As you are present to your breath, your body relaxes and your mind becomes peaceful as the two become joined, integrated. Your experience is whole, here, and now. Breathing in and breathing out. Stay with this focused attention, coming back to your breath whenever your mind wanders, until your timer goes off.

When it does, slowly open your eyes and stretch your body. While still seated, set an intention that you'll walk through your day consciously and attentively. Commit to being with and participating in your daily activities with graceful awareness and presence. Then, throughout the day, be mindful of your breath, which promises to link you to the present moment, the place that offers serenity and freedom. As Thich Nhat Hanh writes, "The present moment is filled with joy and happiness. If you are attentive, you will see it."[22]

Breathing Exercise #3: The Long Exhale (or 1:2 Breathing)

This 1:2 pranayama breathing exercise increases your exhalation gradually, until it's twice the length of your inhalation.

You can practice this exercise just as you turn off the light, or in the middle of the night if you find yourself tossing and turning. As you lengthen your exhale, your breath relaxes your nervous system, calms your mind, and helps you sleep. It's also helpful at any time of day to calm stress or anxiety.

Begin by belly breathing, allowing your belly to rise and fall with each inhalation and exhalation. You can place your palm on your abdomen to experience this rising and falling. Mentally, begin to count the length of each inhalation and exhalation. As you inhale, try counting up to 5. Pause for 1 count. Then exhale for those same 5 counts. Do this for 5 breath cycles. Gradually, begin to lengthen your exhalation by 1 to 2 counts, simply by pulling your abdomen down toward your spine. As long as your breath feels smooth and relaxed, continue to gradually increase the length of your exhalation by 1 to 2 counts once every few breaths.

It's important to feel no strain as your exhalations increase in length. If you feel yourself tensing up or gasping for air, back off. The key is to remain calm. If you can make your exhalation up to twice as long as your inhalations, great. If not—no big deal. Stay with the practice—it will unfold for you just as it's meant to. Even an exhalation that is only slightly longer than the inhalation can induce a calming effect—no need to push yourself beyond your capacity. If you strain, you'll likely feel agitated rather than calm. Complete your practice with 5 to 10 normal breaths.

While the best way to practice pranayama is under the guidance of an experienced teacher, there are simple techniques, such as gentle diaphragmatic breathing and comfortably lengthening the exhalation, that can be used at any time to transform not only your breath, but also your state of mind.

Take a Deep Breath: It's Good for You

Research shows that the practice of deep breathing has specific physiological benefits, such as improving concentration and focus, lowering your blood pressure, strengthening your immune system, and enhancing the functioning of every cell in your body. In a study at the Augusta Women's Center in Augusta, Georgia, researchers showed that pranayama breathing alters your brain's information processing, lowering stress and increasing your sense of well-being. They found that pranayama positively affects immune function, hypertension, asthma, autonomic nervous system imbalances, and psychological or stress-related disorders.[23] Let's take a closer look at a few of these benefits.

Strengthening Your Immune System

Mindful breathing increases the level of oxygen in your body, which increases your energy, fuels every cell, and supports detoxification throughout your entire body. Mladen Golubic, MD, PhD, a physician at the Cleveland Clinic's Center for Lifestyle Medicine and director of the Clinic's Lifestyle 180 program, focuses his research on the breath. Studies among Lifestyle 180 participants, many of whom were unsuccessful traditional disease management programs, reveal that breathing techniques and exercises, along with nutrition and physical activity, significantly improved the health of those with chronic diseases, including obesity, hypertension, hyperlipidemia (high blood fat such as cholesterol and triglycerides), and diabetes. "Breathing can have a profound impact on our physiology and our health," Dr. Golubic says. "You can influence asthma. You can influence chronic obstructive pulmonary disease."[24]

Providing Sufficient Oxygen for Every Cell for Optimal Metabolism

Your cells depend on an "aerobic," or oxygen-rich, environment to function well. Healthy, normal cells require oxygen to metabolize glucose, your cells' primary fuel. With restricted oxygen, you can't metabolize your food properly, nutrients are wasted, and your metabolism becomes a fermentation process, changing the environment of your cells and increasing the likelihood of disease. Cells that are diseased thrive in an oxygen-poor environment. Healthy cells flourish with an abundance of oxygen.

Enhancing Energy Production

Your body uses a chemical called adenosine triphosphate (ATP) to produce energy in your cells in a process called "cellular respiration." Your cells are actually breathing, or taking in air, by taking up oxygen from your blood. Every cell in your body uses oxygen to convert stored glucose into ATP, which, in turn, supplies your body's energy needs. So your breath plays a critical role in supplying your body with energy. If something goes wrong with your production of ATP, the result is lowered vitality, disease, and premature aging.

Improving Focus and Concentration

Most of us breathe from only the top portions of our lungs, which makes our breathing shallow and erratic. But breathing intentionally and deeply provides a steady, soothing flow of oxygen, stabilizing your heart rate, enriching blood oxygen levels, and feeding your brain. When your brain is infused with oxygen, your mood elevates, and you become more focused and tranquil.

In a study at the University of Wisconsin–Madison, 16 participants practiced 3 months of mindfulness meditation training. After each session, they were given an attention task: They were shown a series of letters in rapid succession, then asked to identify the first letter they'd been shown. Among those who participated in mindfulness training, all were able to correctly identify the first letter; among the control group, significantly fewer (16 out of 23) were able to do so. The study showed that 3 months of mindfulness meditation led to a profound shift in the way the brain allocates attention, significantly increasing the brain's ability to focus. The study's lead author, Richard Davidson, says the study confirms that attention is a flexible, trainable skill that can be improved by quieting the mind and performing conscious breathing.[25]

Lowering Blood Pressure

Scientists have determined that a sedentary, stressful lifestyle, combined with high salt intake, reduces your kidneys' ability to rid your body of toxins. Under chronic stress, we tend to take shallow breaths and unconsciously hold them. We know shallow breathing is linked to stress. Shallow breathing also disrupts the blood's chemical balance, creating an acidic state. More acidic blood, in turn, makes your kidneys less efficient at disposing of sodium. Research shows that shallow breathing delays salt excretion enough to raise blood pressure in animals. Dr. David

Anderson, PhD, who heads research on behavior and hypertension at the National Institute on Aging, is testing that same theory on humans. He believes that how we breathe may hold a key to how the body regulates blood pressure—and that it has less to do with relaxation than with breaking down the excessive amount of salt most of us eat.[26]

Since 2002, the Food and Drug Administration has permitted the sale of RESPeRATE, a device that's been designed to help pace breathing in order to lower blood pressure. Clinical trials have shown that those using the device experienced significant drops in their blood pressure.[27]

Anderson is using the same machine to test his own theory: When they're under chronic stress, people tend to breathe high up into their chests, and even hold their breath. Anderson calls this inhibitory breathing. Holding your breath diverts blood to your brain to increase alertness, which helps if you're in danger, but also creates an acidic condition in your blood, rendering your kidneys less efficient at pumping out sodium.[28]

Practice Meditation

Breathing is the basis of meditation, another beneficial technique for detoxing your mind. Remember: What's happening in your mind affects how you feel physically and emotionally—and vice versa. As your breath relaxes, your body releases tension, your mind opens, and your heart softens. Always begin with the breath! It might be helpful to use one of the breathing techniques you've already learned to begin your meditation practice.

Meditation, an ancient practice that's part of many faith traditions, is also used by those who don't practice any religion. It allows practitioners to glimpse their inner nature amid the chaos and distractions of life. There are as many ways to meditate as there are people who engage in the practice. Here's a look at two of the most widely known meditation practices.

Transcendental Meditation

This form of meditation is used to evoke a relaxation response. Practitioners focus on a single "point," usually on the sensation of the breath leaving and entering the body or on a mantra, which might be a special sound or phrase repeated silently. When thoughts or feelings arise, they acknowledge them and go right back to the mantra or single-point attention. These practices, which Buddhists call "Samadhi" or "one-pointed" meditation, can generate a deep sense of calm.

Mindfulness Meditation

Also known as vipassana, or insight meditation, this practice begins by using one-pointed attention to cultivate calmness and stability, then moves beyond that single focus of attention into a broader landscape of observation. When thoughts or feelings rise to the surface in your mind, notice and observe them objectively, moment by moment, as the totality of what's happening here and now. You'll begin to see that thoughts are simply sensory input, and you can begin to be "dispassionate and fundamentally unaffected" by your thoughts, feelings, and external circumstances, as Charlotte Joko Beck, an American Zen teacher, writes in *Everyday Zen*.[29]

The goal of mindfulness is to be more aware of what's happening in the present moment, without judgment, assessment, or manipulation. When you're mindful, you simply notice your thoughts and feelings without reacting to them. If you're experiencing pain or stress, instead of trying to escape from it, try to accept what's happening in the moment— without wishing the moment were different than it is. Be quietly in that moment, knowing that it will change in its own time and engaging in the practice of gratitude for all the moment offers—without holding on to it.

Getting Started

Meditation helps you give up the spinning mind and, even if just for a moment, to simply sit with what is. In the present moment, the mind becomes a bit more still and we are like a mirror, simply seeing everything, reflecting everything. Here are some tips to help you get started or support you in your meditation practice.

Commit to Remaining Open. There's no right or wrong way to meditate and no good or bad meditation. Commit to being open hearted and awake, noticing and accepting everything, judging nothing.

Embrace meditation as an opportunity to connect with your authentic self, with your sincere desire for and capability to achieve love, clarity, and inner peace. Remember: It may be helpful to begin your practice by connecting to your heart's deepest desire. Take a few minutes to determine what matters most to you. You may want to dedicate your practice to your own emotional, mental, and spiritual awakening and freedom, and perhaps extend this blessing to all beings.

Set a Regular Time and Place for Your Meditation. Often, morning is best, because the mind tends to be calmer then. But the best time is the one to which you can realistically and regularly commit, and to decide that, you'll need to determine how long you will sit. Though many choose between 20 and 45 minutes, you might begin with 5 or 10 minutes and work up to an hour. As you establish a habit, you may find you can sit longer and more calmly. Set a timer or choose a meditation app with beautiful ring tones and bells.

If possible, create a quiet space with a favorite chair, cushion, or kneeling bench exclusively for your daily sitting. You may want to add a candle, healing images, photos of loved ones, elements of nature—whatever inspires you.

Sit Up Tall. Keep your spine straight so that your lungs can expand and contract easily with each breath cycle, whether you're on a chair, cushion, or kneeling bench. Be relaxed, alert, open, and receptive, simultaneously. Relax your shoulders and allow your hands to rest comfortably on your knees or lap. In a gesture of receiving, allow your palms to face up to the sky. In a gesture of grounding, turn your palms down on your inner thighs. Let your eyes close. Or, if you prefer, leave your eyes open and gaze softly down a couple of inches beyond your nose.

Stir Your Senses. Take a few minutes to connect with your senses. Listen to the sounds inside and outside the room. Notice the temperature on your skin, the color and texture behind your closed eyelids, and any scent you can detect.

Take a Body Scan, Relaxing with Each Breath. Start with some deep breaths. In an open, relaxed attitude, scan your entire body. First notice your head and feel the sensations there. Then, move your attention downward toward your forehead and eyebrows. Inhale as you soften the lines above your eyebrows. As you exhale, soften behind your eyes. Take your palms to your temples and softly massage them (that's a place we often hold on to tension). Now take your attention down to your jaw. Open your mouth and move your jaw up and down and side to side, releasing any tension. Take your gaze to the back of your neck and shoulders, allowing the tension to slide down your neck and off your fingertips. Inhaling and exhaling, release any tension you're experiencing, physically or emotionally. Slowly relax your entire body, seeking to be open to anything that arises.

Use Your Breath and Your Senses as a Reminder to Return to Presence. When you've drifted off and become lost in thought, don't judge yourself—just gently come back to your breath and relax back into the experience of being right here, right now. Gently recall your attention back to the present. Notice how your breath feels as it enters and leaves your nostrils, and how your belly expands and contracts and your chest rises and falls. You may want to re-relax your forehead, shoulders, hands, and heart, to arrive again with mindful presence to the present moment. With your senses wide awake, you can use any sensation as a reminder to come back gently to the moment.

Practice Nonjudgment/Nonstriving Focused Attention and Concentration. While your attention supports mindfulness, it's important not to strive to achieve anything, from a calm mind to a "good" meditation. Instead, accept and embrace whatever thoughts, feelings, and sensations come up rather than trying to suppress or eliminate them. Try to recognize when you're lost in thought. When you find yourself thinking, planning, or worrying, gently, gracefully, and lovingly bring your attention back to your breath.

Guided Meditation

Guided meditation is simply using a guide to help you practice stillness. It can be a helpful way to enter into meditation. You can do it in a class with a meditation teacher, by listening to a recording, or by using a written guide. If you'd like to try guided meditation, here are some beautiful ways to begin.

Reflective Meditation. Use a poem or spiritual reading that touches your heart. Take one word or line at a time and reflect on it. How does it connect with your life in this present moment? Can you embrace these words for yourself? If not, what gentle, graceful step do you need to take for these words to ring true for you?

Loving-Kindness Meditation. In *A Path with a Heart,*[30] Jack Kornfield offers a guided meditation, based on ancient Tibetan Buddhist practice, that's designed to evoke loving kindness and generosity toward yourself and others. There are many other loving-kindness meditations as well. Here is one to try.

Begin reciting inwardly one or more of the following phrases. Start with loving yourself—without that, it's almost impossible to offer compassion and love toward others.

May I be filled with loving kindness.
May I be well.
May I be peaceful and at ease.
May I be happy.

As you repeat these phrases, picture yourself being held within an open heart of loving kindness and generosity. Adjust the words and images to find the phrases that best open your heart. Repeat those phrases, allowing any contrary feelings—resentment, anger, hurt—to surface. If they do, be patient and kind toward yourself.

When you feel that you've established a sense of loving kindness toward yourself, expand your meditation to include others. Choose someone in your life who has truly cared for you and picture this person as you recite the same phrases: *May (name of person) be filled with loving kindness. . . .* As you express loving kindness toward this person, begin to widen your circle to embrace others you love, picturing each one and reciting the same phrases, evoking a sense of loving kindness for them. Then include others: friends, neighbors, animals, all beings on earth.

May all beings be filled with loving kindness.
May all be well.
May all beings everywhere be peaceful and at ease.
May all beings everywhere be happy.

Now turn your attention to those who have hurt or offended you. Offer them the same loving kindness, sending them healing and peace. Expand your heart from loved ones to all beings everywhere, even those who've caused you harm. It may not all come at once. Be patient with yourself.

Loving kindness can be practiced anywhere, anytime—in the car on your way to work; in long, contentious meetings; in line at the grocery store. This powerful meditation will help you to experience a deeper connection with yourself and others.

Forgiveness and Healing Meditation. When someone has hurt you, consciously or unconsciously, one of the most challenging measures you face is forgiveness—it may seem easier to end the relationship and extricate the offender from your life. But the only way you can ultimately be free is to forgive. If you hold on to resentment, you suffer, but following a path toward forgiveness may lead to freedom from the negative experiences of the past. When you're ready to let go of your own pain, you're able to forgive—but that requires total acceptance of the things that happened and the part we've played.

At the end of your meditation, express your feelings in writing. If you stay with it, you may, like writer Anne Lamott, claim this truth for yourself: "Forgiveness is giving up all hope of having had a different past."[31]

To begin, sit quietly with your eyes closed. Allow your breath to flow in and out, smoothly. Notice the quality of your breath. Now scan your body, bringing your attention to any part that feels tense or tight and using your breath to dissolve the tension. When your mind wanders, take your attention back to your breath.

After a few minutes, take your attention to the crown of your head. Imagine a beautiful glow of loving, living light above you, and feel it streaming light over you. Take this light into the top of your head, onto your forehead, and into your eyes, allowing it to wash your body like a river floods its banks and washes away debris. Allow the light to carry fear, fatigue, anger, resentment, and trauma out through your fingertips and the soles of your feet. As you release these sabotaging feelings, imagine that they are being absorbed by the earth and turned into compost. Embrace this light, whose purpose is to wash and heal your entire body, releasing tension, pain, or hurt. Come back to your breath.

Reflect on what the word *forgiveness* means to you and what forgiveness would look like. Now gently allow the image of someone for whom you harbor resentment to come into your mind. Invite him or her in, very gently, just for this moment. In your heart, practice saying to him or to her:

I forgive you.
I forgive you for whatever you have done that has caused me pain,
intentionally or unintentionally. However you have caused me pain, I
forgive you.

Speak gently in your heart with your own words, in your own way.

Allow the person to be touched, just for the moment, by your forgiveness. Breathe in. Breathe out. Breathe in. Breathe out. Feel your breath. If you can, you may want to offer this blessing:

May you be at peace,
May your heart remain open,
May you awaken to the light of your own true nature,
May you be healed,
May you be a source of healing for all beings.

Now turn your gaze inward, toward yourself. Looking at yourself with the eyes of your heart, silently call yourself by your own first name, and say, I forgive you. I *accept* you completely, just as you are. Let yourself be bathed in this ball of light that is expanding into a circle of light, flooding your heart with love and forgiveness. Offer this blessing to yourself:

May I be at peace,
May my heart remain open,
May I awaken to the light of my own true nature,
May I be healed,
May I be a source of healing for all beings.

Now invite your loved ones into this circle of divine light, calling each of them by name. See them in as much detail as possible, imagining the loving light shining down on them, dispelling darkness, revealing the light within their own hearts. Then bless them:

May you be at peace,
May your heart remain open,
May you awaken to the light of your own true nature,
May you be healed,
May you be a source of healing for all beings.

Extend your gaze further and see the planet as it appears from space. Imagine the earth and all its creatures surrounded by light. Expand your heart wide to hold it all as you offer this blessing:

May there be peace on earth,
May the hearts of all people be open to themselves and to each other,
May they be at peace,
May they be freed of all suffering,
May they be healed,
May all beings be free,
May all people awaken to the light of their own true nature,
May all creation be blessed and be a blessing to all that is.

Take a few moments to rest in the silence of your heart.

Prepare for Restful Sleep

One of the most important ways to support your body's detoxification system is to get sound, deep sleep. During sleep, your liver's detoxifying enzymes are busy at work as your nervous system shifts into its parasympathetic mode and your body redirects its priorities from creating energy and digesting food to detoxifying and rebuilding. During sleep, your liver targets its energy toward breaking down and eliminating carcinogens, and both internal and external toxins. Without sufficient, deep sleep, cleansing and healing are impeded. If you're waking up feeling tired, you may not be getting enough sleep.

Phyllis Zee, MD, PhD, director of the Sleep Disorders Center and the sleep medicine fellowship training program at Northwestern University's Feinberg School of Medicine, studies circadian genes—the "clock genes" contained in every organ in your body.

Dr. Zee is studying the ways sleep deprivation and disturbance affect weight gain. Her findings show the link between eating and sleeping late and an increased risk of weight gain, with the timing of sleep affecting food choices—especially unhealthy ones. Circadian timing and sleep deprivation result in our propensity to eat not only highly processed and fast foods, but to eat at a time of day when our bodies can't process them properly.[32]

Here are some techniques that may help you transition from your workday to sleep time, as well as improve the quality of your sleep. Experiment and see what works best for you.

Turn Off All Screens (iPhone, iPad, computer, TV, etc.) 1 Hour before Sleep. The light from these electronic devices can affect your circadian rhythm, make your brain more awake, and delay sleep.

From a relatively close distance, laptops, iPads, and iPhones directly shine blue light—to which your eyes are especially sensitive. Paper books and many e-book readers, on the other hand, don't emit their own light. Computer screens and phones tend to put out a lot of blue light, which may intensify the screen's stimulating effects.

When receptors in your eyes encounter bright light for an extended time, they send a message to your brain signaling that it's time to be awake. Your brain, in turn, stops secreting melatonin, the hormone that regulates your internal sleep clock. Typically, your brain produces melatonin at about 9 or 10 p.m., but you can fool your brain into stopping melatonin production in the presence of bright lights. To maximize your body's melatonin production, keep iPads and laptops out of the bedroom and shut them down an hour before lights-out.

Take a Bath with Essential Oils and Epsom Salts. Warm, aromatic baths are a soothing way to help relax your body before bedtime. Aromatherapy, using essential oils, can be deliciously relaxing before bed. Lavender, rose, chamomile, and orange are thought to bring a sense of calm and peace to the body and mind at the end of a long day. You'll want to experiment and see which ones feel the most healing to you.

Epsom salts can reduce your body's toxic load by assisting its effort to eliminate toxins through your skin. Epsom salts are simply a salt made of magnesium and sulfate. According to research from the University of Birmingham in England, the salts simultaneously support your liver in its Phase Two detoxification process and soothe your nervous system.[33]

Drink Diaphoretic Teas, which induce perspiration. Try sipping elderberry, yarrow, peppermint, or ginger tea while taking a hot bath. A number of scientific studies show that these perspiration-promoting teas may help you eliminate toxins through your skin and mucous membranes.[34] Soothing teas, such as chamomile, kava kava, lavender, and valerian root can help relax your body and mind for sleep.

Move Your Body. Research shows that the benefits of any kind of movement are more significant than previously known—especially when you move outdoors. In a Japanese study, 20 healthy male volunteers were asked to take a 1,000-meter walk at their own pace, along a mountain path to an observation platform. Forty minutes later, those in the woodland walking group experienced significant decreases in blood pressure, as well as elevated mood and a lower perception of stress.[35] And in a University of Massachusetts study, a group of healthy men were given a 4-inch platform shoe to wear on their right foot so that their left leg was left to dangle above the ground for 2 days. Using crutches, the men never put weight on their left leg. After 2 days, scientists biopsied both legs and found multiple genes being expressed differently in each leg. The conclusion: "Gene activity in the left leg suggested that DNA repair mechanisms had been disrupted, insulin response was dropping, oxidative stress was rising, and metabolic activity within individual muscle cells was slowing only after 48 hours of inactivity."[36] And a study conducted at the Baker IDI Heart and Diabetes Institute in Melbourne, Australia, concluded that any movement, even a 2-minute stroll, every 20 minutes maintained blood sugar levels.[37]

Spend Time in Your Kitchen

Health writer Michael Pollan claims that cooking can change our lives. The best way to take care of our health, he says in his book *Cooked,* is to prepare our own food.[38] Using fresh ingredients connects us to the natural world and strengthens our relationships with family and friends.

When we consume convenience foods, we're relying on corporations to process those foods, which contain large quantities of fat, sugar, and salt. Pollan argues that getting back into the kitchen may be the single most important step to help make our food system healthier and more sustainable.

Though we often avoid cooking because of busy schedules, the gift of cleansing is that it compels us to make time for this healing task. The simple act of preparing food can be both meditative and creative. Chopping, assembling, stirring, serving, and consuming beautiful food requires our presence and stirs our senses, nourishing body, mind, and spirit.

Moving On

In the next chapter, we'll look at one of the most healing practices you can engage in for the health of your mind, body, and spirit—yoga. Even if you've never tried it before, you'll find that the simple moves you'll learn in Chapter 8 are healing and beneficial, and a wonderful accompaniment to your cleanse.

CHAPTER 8

Practicing Wholeness:
Uniting Body and Mind through Yoga

As you journey through your healing cleanse, one of the best things you can do to enhance your experience is to practice yoga. The word, after all, means to yoke—or unite—your mind, body, and spirit, connecting your breath with movement and meditation. According to B. K. S. Iyengar, one of the world's foremost yoga teachers, yoga stills the restlessness of the mind, the intellect, and the self.[1] In yoking your breath with the physical practice or *asana,* a Sanskrit word that means to sit in a yoga posture, your body relaxes and your mind quiets in preparation for seated meditation.

Yoga is particularly supportive while cleansing because, as we're learning, it calms your sympathetic nervous system, suppressing your stress response by reducing your cortisol levels. Thirty-one musicians at the Tanglewood Music Center, the summer home of the Boston Symphony in Lennox, Massachusetts, participated in an 8-week study examining the effects of yoga on stress. Compared with a control group, those who took part in yoga sessions experienced lower performance-related anxiety as well as an overall improvement in mood.[2]

Science also shows that yoga stimulates your parasympathetic nervous system (PNS), which calms you down after a stress trigger. When your parasympathetic nervous system is aroused, your body directs blood toward your endocrine glands, digestive organs, and lymphatic system, while lowering your heart rate and blood pressure. With the parasympathetic nervous system in gear, your body can use nutrients—and eliminate toxins—more effectively.[3]

The practice of yoga gives you time and space to pause, encouraging you to focus your attention within the boundaries of your mat. There, your goal is to find the rhythm of your breath and link it to the flow of movement from one pose to another. The beauty of yoga is that it's non-competitive and available to everyone, at any age and any level of fitness. Yoga requires no special equipment, and you can practice it anywhere. In fact, your yoga practice is always with you, as close as your breath and your body.

Through the practice of pranayama (controlled breathing; see the exercises in Chapter 7) and movement, yoga increases your strength, your energy, and your ability to relax while simultaneously helping relieve tension and reduce stress, creating balanced wellness within. But just how does it work?

In yoga, your strength comes from your breath and your core, the abdominal muscles that support your organs and limbs. While your breath is strengthening your body, it simultaneously energizes and relaxes you.

This is the way it works: Your cells, tissues, organs, and muscles need oxygen to produce energy and to function well. Your limbs need the strength of your core muscles to stabilize, align, and move freely. When you move from your core, you improve your physical and mental performance while protecting yourself from injury. Strengthening your body increases your energy, sharpens your focus, and improves your physical and mental endurance. While yoga is like other forms of exercise, in that it engages your breath and concentration, it's also different in some important ways.

Scientists at Duke University Medical Center reviewed more than 100 studies on the effects of yoga on a variety of major psychiatric disorders. After narrowing their field to the highest-quality studies, they chose 16 to focus on and found that yoga holds benefits for disorders ranging from sleep complaints and ADHD to schizophrenia and depression.[4] Their research revealed that yoga:

- Increases serotonin levels
- Reduces inflammation
- Reduces oxidative stress
- Enhances mental health

Science is proving what yoga practitioners have always known: When you inhale deeply, you infuse your body with high-octane fuel, invigorating your cells to reduce oxidation and inflammation. When you exhale, you release tension, lowering emotional and mental stress. By linking conscious breath to movement, yoga can increase your energy and shift your mind, providing an authentic emotional, mental, and spiritual detox while cultivating a quiet mind, a balanced body, and a renewed spirit.

If you're new to yoga—or if you've been away from the practice— these poses will help you get started. You can practice one pose at a time or attempt to link a few together until you are ready to practice the whole sequence at one time.

Each time you practice, begin with an acceptance of your body and yourself. Give yourself time to relax by focusing on your breath. From there, allow your body to release and open naturally. From this acceptance—and your willingness to cooperate with your body, rather than fight against it—you'll find balance, serenity, and peace in your body, mind, and spirit. And as you commit to a regular practice on your mat, you'll begin to notice that you feel more balanced and peaceful off your mat too.

Cleansing Yoga Poses

There are hundreds of yoga poses, or *asanas*, that strengthen, detox, and balance your body; calm and clear your mind; and open your heart. As you pursue a regular practice, you'll notice more flexibility and stability in your body, more space and freedom in your mind, and more peace and compassion in your heart.

Here are a few poses, linked together by your breath. Honor yourself and your journey, and remember to be gentle with yourself. You don't have to accomplish it all in one day.

SUN SALUTATION A (SURYA NAMASKARA)

Sun Salutation is a warming and energizing series of poses, alternating forward bends and backbends in a fluid sequence. As its name implies, Sun Salutation was traditionally practiced while facing east to welcome the morning. These poses tone your inner organ ring (liver, pancreas, spleen, kidneys), stretch your low back and hamstrings, strengthen your abdominal and back muscles, develop upper body strength, and activate energy that grounds you to the earth.

At the beginning of your yoga practice, Sun Salutation A builds heat. Throughout your practice, these poses allow you to reset your body and mind. The sequence of movements, linked by breath, between various poses is often called a "connecting vinyasa." Traditionally, this sequence involves one breath per movement and lets the body and mind reset. If you're a beginner, you can take as many breaths between each pose as necessary. In this sample sequence, a connecting vinyasa is offered between poses. Take what you need and leave the rest. If you'd like, take one pose and try it on both sides, skipping the vinyasa.

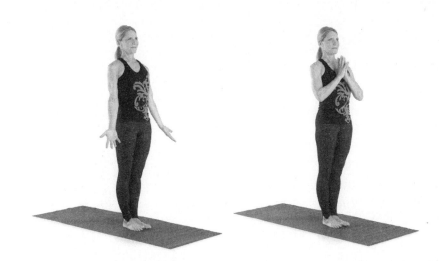

MOUNTAIN OR STANDING POSE (*TADASANA*)

Learning how to stand is the foundation of your practice and your relationship to the ground, to gravity, and to your spine. Mountain Pose is the most important pose, providing fundamental alignment and stability. When your feet and legs ground you properly and your pelvis is neutral, you give your upper body the strength and confidence to be light and agile. Proper spinal alignment allows energy to flow freely, invigorating your body, mind, and spirit.

In this pose, your spine lengthens while your torso, chest, and shoulders open. Just as trees and plants send roots down into the earth and branches up to the sky, you will press your feet to the earth and rise tall.

• Begin by standing with your feet hip-width apart.

• Press into all four corners of your feet. Lift your toes. Drive your legs and feet down into the earth. Lift your chest to lengthen your spine while rooting your lower body down.

• Find neutral pelvis by rocking it forward and backward, tucking your tailbone under and then sending your tailbone back. Rock your pelvis back and forth to see if you can find a place right in the middle, a place that feels "just right," where your pelvis is just floating.

• Pull the tops of your shoulders back and broaden your shoulder blades across your back.

• Allow your arms to hang by your sides, palms facing forward, in a gesture of receiving.

• Gaze forward. Stand like a mountain.

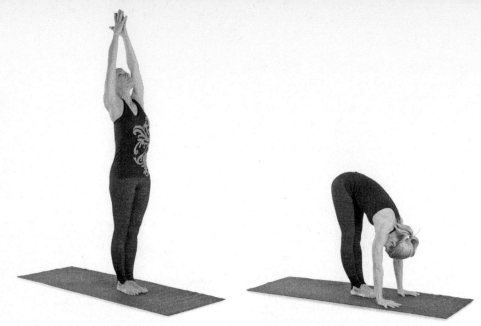

UPWARD-FACING HANDS POSE (*URDHVA HASTASANA*)

This pose opens your torso, neck, chest, and shoulders. With hands overhead, this pose relieves gravitational compression on your body.

• From Mountain Pose, inhale as you sweep your arms up, and out to the sides, reaching overhead, shoulder-width apart. If comfortable, bring your palms together.

• Straighten your elbows if possible.

• Take your gaze upward.

STANDING FORWARD FOLD (*UTTANASANA*)

Standing Forward Fold Pose is a resting pose for your heart, because when you're in it, your head is below your heart. Use the pose to stretch and relax your upper body. Like all inversions, it clears and balances your mind. If your hamstrings are tight or your lower back is weak, bend your knees softly.

• From *Urdhva Hastasana*, hingeing at the hips you fold forward, bringing your palms to the ground.

• Press your chest toward your thighs and bring your chin toward your shins.

• Draw the crown of your head down toward the mat. Allow your neck to be long.

• If your palms don't reach the mat, put a soft bend in your knees.

Take this pose twice more, resting for 2 breath cycles in between.

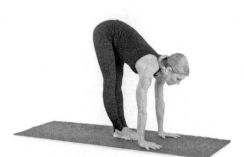

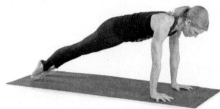

HALF FORWARD FOLD
(*ARDHA UTTANASANA*)

Half Forward Fold stretches your hamstrings, elongates your spine, and engages your abdominals.

• From Standing Forward Fold, keep your fingertips on the mat. Inhale as you lift your torso halfway up, keeping your back flat and neck long, bending your knees if necessary. If your hamstrings are tight, you can also bring your palms to your shins.

• Bend your knees as much as you need in order to keep your back flat.

• Gaze at a spot on the floor 6 inches ahead of your toes.

HIGH PUSHUP (PLANK)

This pose builds both upper and lower body strength while coordinating and integrating the entire musculoskeletal system. Plank pose strengthens your abdominals, chest, arms, and legs.

• From Half Forward Fold, exhale as you step back so that you are at the top of a pushup.

• Stand on the balls of your feet.

• Stack your shoulders over your wrists, spread your shoulder blades apart, and pull them down your back.

• Lift your kneecaps up to engage your quadriceps (thighs).

• Draw your navel up to your spine and hollow out your belly.

• Set your gaze between your thumbs to lengthen your neck.

• If this pose places too much strain on your shoulders, wrists, or core, lower your knees to the mat, keeping a straight line from your knees to the crown of your head.

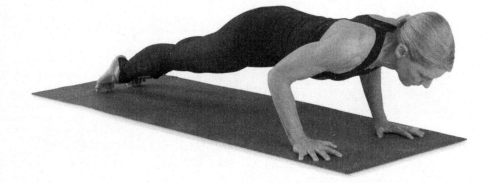

LOW PUSHUP (*CHATURANGA DANDASANA*)

Low Pushup contracts your core abdominals, releases your low back, and develops your upper body strength. This pose engages the entire musculature, activating and developing a connection between your core, your legs and feet, and your arms and hands. It can be challenging for those just beginning to practice. In that case, lower your knees to the mat for a modified Low Pushup.

• From High Pushup, exhale and bend your elbows, drawing them backward close beside your ribs.

• As you lower your torso toward the floor, move your upper body forward, and hover over the mat until your elbows are bent at 90 degrees.

• Draw your navel to your spine and hollow out your belly.

• Hug your elbows in by your sides and pull your shoulders away from your ears.

• Gaze forward.

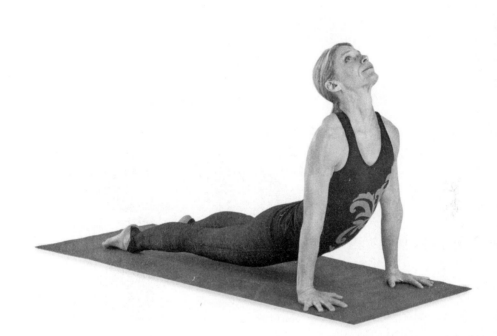

UPWARD-FACING DOG (*URDHVA MUKHA SVANASANA*)

Upward-Facing Dog prepares your body for back-bending poses. It lengthens your spine and strengthens your back and arms, while expanding your entire front torso.

• From Low Pushup, inhale, press down on your hands, and scoop your chest forward.

• As you lift your torso up, roll over the tops of your toes and move your torso forward.

• Press the tops of your feet down into the mat.

• Engage your quadriceps to lift the tops of your thighs off the mat.

• Pull your shoulders down your back, squeezing them together, as you press your chest forward and up.

• Gaze forward so that your neck is in line with your spine.

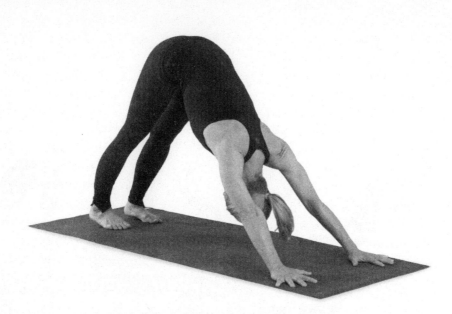

DOWNWARD-FACING DOG (*ADHO MUKHA SVANASANA*)

Downward-Facing Dog is one of the most important poses in yoga, connecting your body, mind, and spirit. It lengthens your spine, extends your legs, strengthens your ankles, and develops your upper body and leg strength, while easing stiffness in your neck, shoulders, and wrists. Downward-Facing Dog calms your nervous system, engages your abdominals, and stretches your hamstrings (the muscles in the backs of your thighs). Holding this pose reduces fatigue, restores energy, and calms your nervous system, creating grounding energy in both your hands and feet simultaneously.

• From Upward-Facing Dog, exhale, curl your toes, and lift your sits bones high to the sky, creating an inverted V with your body.

• Pull your shoulders away from your ears, then spread them out, and roll them down your back.

• Press your palms flat and spread your fingers wide. If your wrists begin to ache, press the knuckles of your index fingers down to balance your weight and protect your wrists.

• Contract your quadriceps to redistribute your weight onto your legs and off of your wrists.

• Draw your navel up and press it back to your spine. Hollow out your belly.

• Take your gaze up to your thighs or navel, if you can.

• Remain in Downward-Facing Dog for 5 complete breath cycles, inhaling and exhaling with long, fluid breaths.

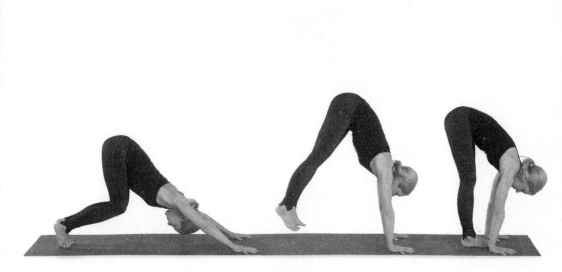

STEP, JUMP, OR FLOAT FORWARD TO COMPLETE SUN SALUTATION A

This motion links one pose to another and brings your feet back to the top of your mat.

• After 5 breath cycles in Downward-Facing Dog, inhale and exhale one more time. As you exhale, press all the air out, lift your heels, bend your knees, and press your thighbones back.

• As you inhale, look at your hands and, using your abdominal muscles, shift your weight onto your hands and spring your feet forward to the top of your mat. If this doesn't work for you, walk your feet to the top of the mat for Standing Forward Fold. Exhale.

• From Standing Forward Fold, inhale. Lift halfway up with a straight back to Half Forward Fold.

• Exhale and fold forward, hinging at your hips, to arrive in Standing Forward Fold with fingertips pressing into the mat.

• From here, use your abdominals to lift and lengthen your torso as you sweep to standing on an inhalation, extending your arms overhead to Upward-Facing Hands. Bring your palms together.

• From Upward-Facing Hands, exhale and bring your arms down by your sides for Mountain Pose. Relax your shoulders down your back and away from your ears. Soften your gaze.

• Repeat Sun Salutation A 2 to 5 times.

SUN SALUTATION B (*SURYA NAMASKAR B*)

Sun Salutation B is a second series of poses that continue warming and energizing your body. It includes several of the poses from Sun Salutation A, plus a few additional ones.

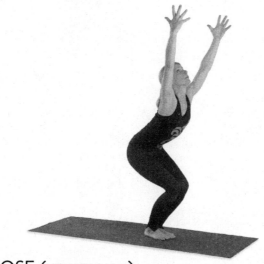

CHAIR POSE (*UTKATASANA*)

Chair Pose is an energizing pose, stimulating your heart, diaphragm, and abdominal organs. This vigorous pose lengthens your spine, releases your low back, opens your shoulders, and engages your quadriceps. It is a big confidence builder.

• From Mountain Pose, inhale as you bend your knees and sweep your arms overhead, bringing your biceps next to your ears with your palms facing each other.

• Squat down and sit back, as if you're sitting down on a kindergarten chair. Sit down low.

• Lift your toes and shift the majority of your weight back to your heels.

• Lift your sternum.

• Spread your shoulder blades apart and rotate your pinky fingers forward and down, so that your thumbs are facing up. Reach your fingertips high.

• If your neck allows you to do so comfortably, look up through your hands.

• Hold the pose for 3 to 5 breath cycles.

I've included connecting vinyasas but please feel free to skip any or all. They're always optional.

CONNECTING VINYASA

A connecting vinyasa is a series of three or four poses from Sun Salutation that helps reestablish long, fluid breathing. It includes these poses: High Pushup (Plank), Low Pushup, Upward-Facing Dog, and Downward-Facing Dog.

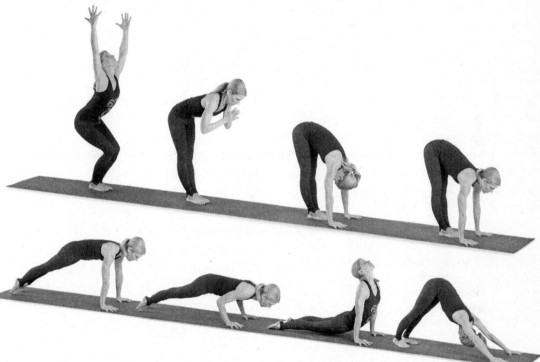

• After your 5th breath in Chair Pose, exhale as you fold forward, hinging at your hips.

• Come into Standing Forward Fold.

• From Forward Fold, inhale and lift halfway to Half Forward Fold.

• Exhale through Forward Fold, stepping back to High Pushup.

• Continue to exhale as you lower down halfway to Low Pushup.

• Inhale to Upward-Facing Dog.

• Exhale and lift your hips high as you move into Downward-Facing Dog.

• Hold the pose for 5 breath cycles.

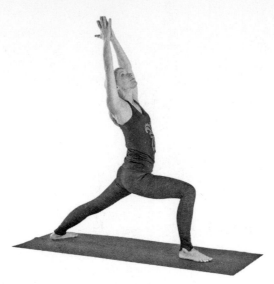

WARRIOR I (*VIRABHADRASANA I*)

As the name implies, Warrior poses are based on fighting stances, similar to those in martial arts. This pose strengthens your legs, opens your shoulders, and activates your entire body in preparation for back bends. Your lower body provides strength and stability, while your upper body is active, light, and open.

WARRIOR I—RIGHT SIDE

• From Downward-Facing Dog, inhale. Pivot your left foot, keeping it flat and turning your toes out 45 degrees. Exhale as you step your right foot forward, bending your knee until it forms a 90-degree angle.

• With your heels in line with one another, square your hips, pulling your left hip back and your right hip forward. You may want to take the outer edges of your feet to the outer edges of your mat so you can square your hips more easily.

• Inhale. Sweep your arms overhead with your palms facing each other and pinky fingers rotated inward, as in Chair Pose.

• Gaze at a nonmoving spot straight ahead, or take your gaze to your thumbs.

• Hold for 5 breath cycles.

CONNECTING VINYASA

• From Warrior I, exhale and take your hands down flat on the mat on either side of your front foot.

• Step your right foot back to High Pushup position.

• Follow Sun Salutation A: Continue to exhale as you lower down to Low Pushup.

• Inhale up to Upward-Facing Dog.

• Exhale back to Downward-Facing Dog.

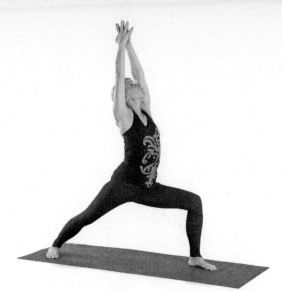

WARRIOR I—LEFT SIDE

• From Downward-Facing Dog, exhale. Pivot your right foot, keeping it flat and turning your toes out 45 degrees. Step your left foot forward, bending your knee until it forms a 90-degree angle.

• With your heels in line with one another, square your hips, pulling your right hip back and your left hip forward. Again, if it's helpful, separate your feet to either edge of the mat in order to open your hips a bit more easily.

• Inhale. Sweep your arms overhead with your palms facing each other and pinky fingers rotated inward, as in Chair Pose.

• Gaze at a nonmoving spot straight ahead, or take your gaze to your thumbs.

• Breathe for 5 breath cycles.

CONNECTING VINYASA

• From Warrior I, exhale and take your hands down flat on the mat on either side of your front foot.

• Step your left foot back to High Pushup.

• Continue to exhale as you lower down to Low Pushup.

• Inhale, pressing up to Upward-Facing Dog.

• Exhale, lift your hips high, and go back to Downward-Facing Dog.

• Take 5 deep inhalations and exhalations. On the 5th breath, exhale completely; as you inhale, jump or walk your feet toward your hands.

• Exhale into Forward Fold.

• Inhale into Chair Pose, sweeping your arms overhead and bending your knees. Hold Chair Pose for a few breaths. Exhale as you rise into Mountain Pose drawing your hands to your heart.

• Repeat Sun Salutation B a few more times.

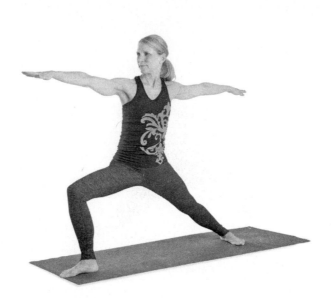

WARRIOR II (*VIRABHADRASANA II*)

Warrior II opens your hips and engages your quadriceps, abdominals, and buttocks. Like Warrior I, Warrior II strengthens your legs, opens your shoulders, and activates your entire body. This pose calms your mind in that it requires concentration and focus to hold the pose in correct alignment.

WARRIOR II—RIGHT SIDE

• From Downward-Facing Dog, inhale, stepping your right foot forward and lifting your torso into Warrior I. From Warrior I, exhale and open your arms out (parallel with your shoulders and the ground) as you open your chest and hips to the side. Turn your palms down as your arms stay lifted.

• You may need to readjust your stance. (You want to take the full length of the mat with your feet in this pose.)

• Heel-toe your front foot out just a bit, so it's in line with the arch in your back foot.

• Press down on the outer edge of your back foot as you bend your front knee to a 90-degree angle, bringing your front thigh parallel to the floor.

• Keep your back toes turned out at 45 degrees from the front of your mat.

• Fix your gaze just beyond the middle finger on your right hand.

• Hold for 5 breath cycles.

• Take Warrior II to the left side if you're not moving on to Reverse Warrior.

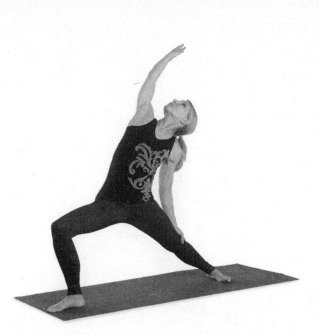

REVERSE WARRIOR (*VIPARITA VIRABHADRASANA*)

Reverse Warrior Pose maintains the strong base of Warrior II, while introducing a side bend. As the front side of your body extends backward, this pose offers a counterpose to Downward-Facing Dog.

REVERSE WARRIOR—RIGHT SIDE

• From Warrior II, exhale and drop your back (left) hand to the back of your left thigh. Flip your front (right) palm up to face the ceiling. Inhale and sweep your front arm overhead.

• Inhale and reach your right arm up to the ceiling, bringing your biceps toward your right ear.

• Bending back slightly, attempting to take your gaze up to your lifted hand.

• Hold for 3 breath cycles.

• Take Reverse Warrior to the left side if you're not moving on to Triangle Pose.

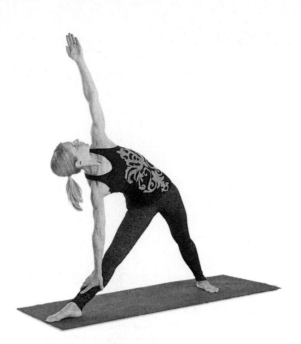

TRIANGLE (*UTTHITA TRIKONASANA*)

Triangle Pose strengthens your legs, creates flexibility in your hips, and relieves tension in your back. The pose is grounding and expansive at the same time.

TRIANGLE—RIGHT SIDE

• From Reverse Warrior, inhale. Come back up to Warrior II by bringing both arms out wide in line with your shoulders with your palms down. Exhale.

• From Warrior II, inhale and straighten your front leg.

• Reach and stretch your front arm out in front of you, lengthening the right side of your body. As you exhale, bring your fingertips down to your shin.

• Inhale, lifting your left arm up toward the sky with your palm open and facing the same direction as your chest. Gaze toward your raised hand. If this is painful for your neck, look down at your right toe.

• Stack your left shoulder on top of your right.

• Tuck your tailbone and your belly so your entire body is in one plane.

• Hold for 5 breath cycles.

• Take Triangle to the left side if you're not moving on to the connecting vinyasa.

CONNECTING VINYASA

• Inhale, coming back to Warrior II by bending your front knee and bringing your arms out wide, parallel with your shoulders, with your palms down.

• From Warrior II, exhale and rotate your arms down, framing your front foot with your palms.

• Continue to exhale as you step back to High Pushup.

• Continue exhaling as you lower down to Low Pushup.

• Inhale up to Upward-Facing Dog.

• Exhale back to Downward-Facing Dog.

• Hold for 5 breath cycles.

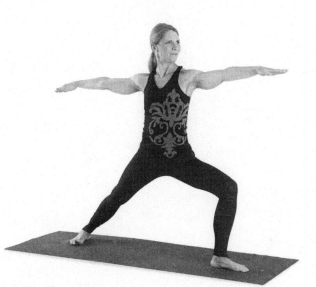

WARRIOR II—LEFT SIDE

• From Downward-Facing Dog, inhale. Step your left foot forward, pivot your right foot out 45 degrees, and sweep your arms overhead for Warrior I Pose.

• Exhale and open your arms to Warrior II, opening your chest and hips to the side.

• Turn your palms down as your arms stay lifted, parallel with your shoulders.

• Press down on the outer edge of your back foot as you bend your front knee to a 90-degree angle, bringing your front thigh parallel to the floor.

• Fix your gaze just beyond the middle finger on your left hand.

• Hold for 5 breath cycles.

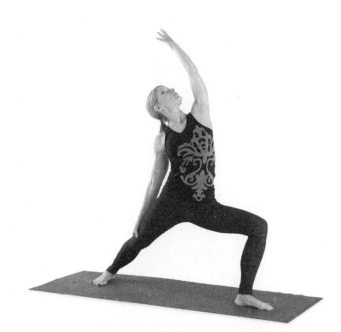

REVERSE WARRIOR—LEFT SIDE

• From Warrior II, exhale. Drop your back (right) hand to the back of your right thigh. Flip your front (left) palm up to face the ceiling.

• Inhale and reach your left arm up to the ceiling, bringing your left bicep right by your left ear.

• Bending back slightly, take your gaze up to your lifted hand.

• Take your gaze up to your lifted hand.

• Hold for 3 breath cycles.

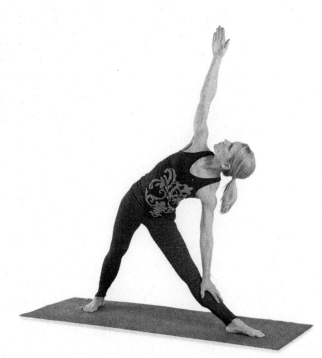

TRIANGLE—LEFT SIDE

• From Reverse Warrior, inhale and come back up to Warrior II by bringing both arms out wide, in line with your shoulders with your palms down. Exhale.

• From Warrior II, inhale and straighten your front leg.

• Reach and stretch your front (left) arm out in front of you, lengthening the left side of your body. As you exhale, lower your left fingertips down to your shin.

• Inhale and lift your right arm up toward the sky with your palm open and facing the same direction as your chest. Gaze toward your raised hand. If this is painful for your neck, look down at your right toe.

• Stack your right shoulder on top of your left.

• Tuck your tailbone and your belly so your entire body is in one plane.

• Hold for 5 breath cycles.

CONNECTING VINYASA

• Inhale, coming back to Warrior II by bending your front knee and bringing your arms out wide, parallel with your shoulders, with your palms turned down.

• From Warrior II, exhale and rotate your arms down, framing your front foot with your palms.

• Continue to exhale as you step back to High Pushup.

• Follow Sun Salutation A: Continue exhaling as you lower down to Low Pushup.

• Inhale up to Upward-Facing Dog.

• Exhale back to Downward-Facing Dog.

• Hold for 5 breath cycles.

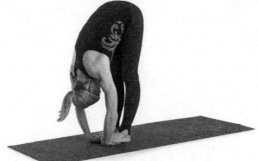

HANDS-TO-FEET POSE (*PADAHASTASANA*)

Hands-to-Feet Pose is a deep forward bend that releases your back and serves as a reset button for your body and mind. Forward folds create balance in your body and mind, allowing you to come back to center in a calm state of concentration.

• From Downward-Facing Dog, walk your hands back to your feet. (If you're doing this pose by itself, begin by getting into Standing Forward Fold.)

• Grasp your big toes with your thumbs, index, and middle fingers, palms facing inward. If possible, slide your palms under your feet until your toes reach the insides of your wrists. Bend your knees as much as you need to in order to bring your ribs close to your thighs.

• As you inhale, lift halfway up.

• As you exhale, hinge at your hips and fold forward, bringing your weight forward toward the balls of your feet.

• Use the strength of your arms and upper body to pull your torso down, bringing your chin toward your shins.

• Slowly begin to straighten your knees only as much as you can while keeping your ribs close to your thighs. If straightening your knees pulls your hamstrings, keep your knees bent.

• Set your gaze behind you.

• Hold for 5 breath cycles.

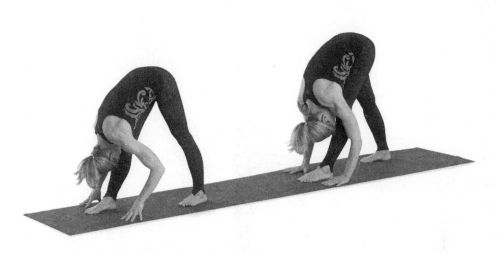

PYRAMID POSE (*PARSVOTTANASANA*)

Pyramid Pose is a deep stretch that strengthens your legs, expands and elongates your hamstrings, stimulates your inner organs through compression, and clears your head.

• From Hands-to-Feet Pose, release your big toes. If your palms are under your feet, lift your toes and slide your palms out. Inhale and sweep your arms all the way up as you rise into Upward-Facing Hands, standing with arms overhead. (If you're doing this pose by itself, begin in Mountain Pose.)

• Exhale, bringing your hands to your waist.

• Step your left foot back one leg length. Keep your heels at least hip-width apart so you can square your hips to the front.

• Inhale and lift your chest, bringing your elbows toward each other behind your back. Exhale and hinge forward from your waist, twisting slightly to bring your navel over your front thigh.

• Bring your hands to the floor or to your front shin, if your hamstrings are tight.

• Gaze toward your back foot and bring the crown of your head toward your front foot.

• Hold the pose for 5 breath cycles.

• Come up to standing and repeat the pose on the opposite side. Hold the pose on the opposite side for 5 breath cycles. At the end of those 5 breath cycles, bring your hands to the mat, framing your front foot. Step both feet back to Downward-Facing Dog, or take a connecting vinyasa, ending with Downward-Facing Dog.

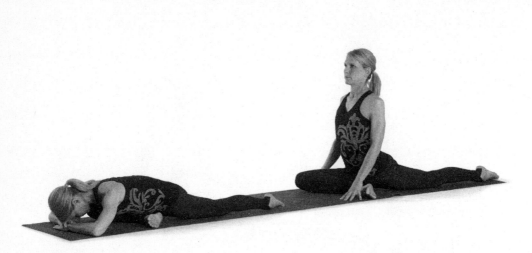

ONE-LEGGED KING PIGEON POSE (*EKA PADA RAJAKAPOTASANA*)

One-Legged Pigeon Pose is a hip-opening pose that releases the piriformis muscle, which attaches the outside of each hip to the sacrum (the lowest section of your spine). The piriformis engages to turn your leg outward. It is one of the most commonly irritated muscles in the body and can cause pain. When it tightens, it can pinch the sciatic nerve, which runs through and under the piriformis muscle, triggering pain in your buttocks and down your leg.

• From Downward-Facing Dog, inhale and lift your right leg up.

• Exhale and draw your right leg forward, bending your right knee and placing it on the mat just behind your right wrist.

• Inhale and slide your left leg straight back in line with your left hip. Squaring your hips, rotate your inner thigh upward, so that you're on top of your left leg.

• Begin with a deep bend in your right knee and your heel close to the left side of your groin.

• Exhale. Fold forward with a flat back, hinging from your waist. Stretch your arms out in front of you.

• Inhale, lengthening your spine. Exhale and bring your forehead to the mat.

• Stay in the pose for 1 full minute. Notice your right hip opening. Breathe into that space, releasing any tightness you feel.

• Inhale, walking your palms back by your sides. Pressing into your palms, lift your hips to sweep your right leg back. Lift your left knee off the mat; come into Downward-Facing Dog.

• Repeat on your left side, holding the pose for 1 full minute.

CONNECTING VINYASA

• From Downward-Facing Dog, inhale, and glide to Plank by bringing your shoulders over your wrists and your hips in line with your shoulders. Exhale as you lower yourself all the way down to the mat.

• Resting on your belly, bring your arms by your sides, palms up, with your cheek to the mat.

• Hold for 5 full breath cycles.

LOCUST POSE (*SALABHASANA*)

Locust Pose is a gentle back-bending pose that strengthens all the musculature of your back while lengthening and opening the front of your body. With your inner organs against the mat, Locust Pose gives these organs a detoxifying massage.

• If you're not already lying facedown on the mat, lie down with your arms by your sides, palms up.

• Bring your chin to the floor.

• Separate your feet so they are hip-width apart.

• Inhale, and in one fluid motion, lift your arms, chest, ribs, thighs, and feet off the floor. Keep your legs straight and active, sending energy through the balls of your feet.

• Reach the crown of your head toward the wall in front of you, so your neck is long and in line with your spine.

• Inhale. Extend your chest forward.

• Exhale. Extend your legs back and up.

• Pull your shoulders away from your ears.

• Hold the pose for 3 breath cycles.

• Lower all the way down.

• Place the opposite cheek on the mat. Breathe for 5 breath cycles.

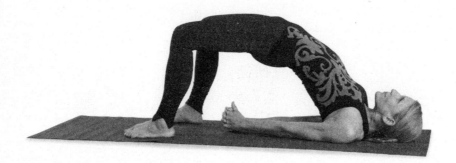

BRIDGE POSE (*SETU BANDHASANA*)

Bridge Pose maintains the energizing effects of Locust Pose, bringing life-giving energy prana to your entire body while bringing awareness to your spine.

• Roll over onto your back with your arms by your sides, palms facing down.

• Bend your knees and place your feet flat on the floor, hip-width apart.

• Bend your elbows so your fingers are pointing toward the ceiling, palms facing toward each other.

• Tilt your pelvis up and scoop your tailbone under.

• Inhale as you lower your forearms to the mat. Lift your hips up high, coming onto your shoulders.

• Walk your shoulder blades in toward each other, underneath your torso, and interlace your fingers with palms together.

• Press down through the soles of your feet and your upper arms as you lift your hips high.

• Lift your chin away from your heart center, pressing your heart high. Hold for 5 breath cycles or 1 minute.

• Release your hands and lower your hips to the mat, rolling down your spine, one vertebra at a time.

• Take 2 deep breaths.

• Take this pose twice more, resting for 2 breath cycles in between.

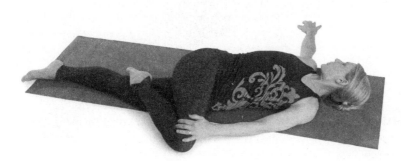

SUPINE TWIST (*SUPTA MATSYENDRASANA*)

As a closing pose, Supine Twist wrings out toxins in your inner organs and releases any remaining tension in your lower spine. It allows you to release anything you might still be holding, creating calm and balance in your body, mind, and spirit.

• Lying on your back with your legs out straight, pull your right knee in toward your right armpit.

• Exhale and drop your right knee over to the outer left side of your body.

• Extend your right arm out straight, parallel to your right shoulder, and look over your right shoulder.

• Place your left hand on your right knee.

• Inhale. Breathe in cleansing, rejuvenating prana.

• On your exhalation, take your attention to your entire spine and release any tension you may be holding. Bathe your spine with your inhalations and exhalations.

Stay here for 1 minute.

• With your left leg out straight, notice your spine wringing out any remaining tension and stress. Twists tone and purify your abdominal organs and kidneys.

• Bring your right leg back to center. Reverse sides, and take another minute in the pose on the left side.

• Notice any tightness or tension on your left side. Breathe out and release, letting go of anything that is not serving you.

• Return to center, hug your knees to your chest, and then release both legs down to the floor for your last pose, Savasana.

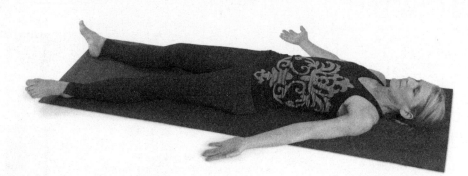

CORPSE POSE (*SAVASANA*)

This final resting pose is the most important pose of your entire practice. In fact, many yogis would argue that your asana practice, the physical practice, is merely preparation for Savasana and meditation. This pose relaxes your physical body and calms your entire being by releasing unconscious tension. As preparation for meditation, Savasana calms your mind while developing full awareness. Your mind will be at peace yet highly alert. Your heart will be open and full. This place of stillness increases vitality and emotional stability while reducing stress and negative emotions.

• While lying on your mat, close your eyes. Place your arms by your sides, palms up.

• Allow your feet to flop out. Feel the strength of the floor holding the entire backside of your body. Allow your body to melt into the floor.

• Let your breath come into its natural rhythm.

• Breathe and let go.

• If your lower back is sore, bend your knees and let the soles of your feet rest on the floor. You can roll up a blanket or towel and place it under your knees.

• Stay in this pose as long as you prefer, allowing all the benefits of your practice to be absorbed into your body, mind, and spirit. The longer you rest, the more healing you bring to your entire being.

• When you're ready, and with your eyes still closed, roll over onto your right side and pause. Using your arms to lift you, rise up. Come to a seated position, bringing your hands into prayer position at your heart center.

• Close your practice by quietly saying "Namaste," which means, "The light in me sees and acknowledges the light in you."

Now you're ready for meditation.

The LiverUp! Diaries

SALLY STEPHENSON, 46

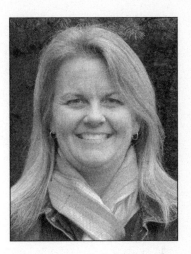

Healthier and Happier

Migraines: From frequent to rare

Lost: 12 pounds

Belly: Flat at last

Migraines used to be a nightmare for me. They'd come out of nowhere—I'd throw up and be in misery for hours. They'd be completely debilitating. I couldn't just lie on the couch until they passed—that'd make things worse—so I'd take a walk. Sometimes that helped, sometimes it didn't.

A couple of years ago, I decided to try the LiverUp! Cleanse, just because I was interested in trying something that sounded so pure and healthy. But the very first day of the cleanse, I got a horrible migraine—one of my worst ever. I went to bed that night thinking that I'd just give up the cleanse the next morning.

But the funny thing was, the next morning, the migraine was gone and I felt better than ever. And it's pretty much stayed that way. My once-a-month migraines have decreased to just once or twice a year. I really think it was the cleanse that changed everything. It taught me a whole new way of eating and showed me the best things to put into my body. I learned that I have triggers that can bring on a migraine—red wine and even dehydration are sometimes triggers for an attack. During the cleanse, of course, you don't have any alcohol and you drink tons of water, and I found that my body really responded to this new way of eating.

I wasn't really heavy before, though I could have stood to lose a few pounds. But during the cleanse, weight came off so quickly—I lost a pound a day, for a total of 12 pounds, and my stomach was flat again. It was amazing.

The cleanse changed the way I look at food and gave me so many new foods to try with my family. It gave me so much energy—I felt awake and clear-headed all the time, and I think I even slept better at night. I was health-conscious before the cleanse, but this brought me to a whole new level. For me, it was absolutely life changing.

CHAPTER 9

Delicious, Healing Recipes

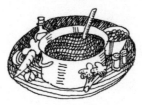

BREAKFAST

SALADS

MAIN MEALS

FRUIT AND SMOOTHIES

Kale Muffins

Prep Time: 15 minutes • Total Time: 35 minutes   Makes 12

1 cup almond flour	1 banana, mashed
1 cup rolled oats, ground	1 cup plain cultured coconut yogurt
½ cup ground flax seeds	¼ cup coconut oil
1 tablespoon baking soda	1 cup coconut milk (from carton) or apple juice
¼ teaspoon cinnamon	2 cups finely chopped kale
3 eggs	2 carrots, shredded

1. Preheat the oven to 375°F. Line a 12-cup muffin pan with unbleached paper liners.

2. In a large bowl, combine the almond flour, oats, flax seeds, baking soda, and cinnamon.

3. In a blender, combine the eggs, banana, yogurt, oil, coconut milk or apple juice, kale, and carrots. Blend until smooth. Pour into the oat mixture and stir to combine. If batter is too dry, add more coconut milk or apple juice until ingredients fold and blend fully.

4. Divide the batter among the muffin cups. Bake for 20 to 25 minutes, or until a wooden pick inserted into the center of a muffin comes out clean. Remove from the pan and cool completely on a rack.

TIP: *A heavy-duty blender, such as a Vitamix, or a food processor will make quick work of shredding the carrots and grinding the oats. For variety, you can add raisins, berries, or nuts to the batter.*

Per serving (1 muffin): 200 calories, 7 g protein, 15 g carbohydrates, 14 g total fat, 6 g saturated fat, 4 g fiber, 348 mg sodium

Spinach and Mushroom Omelet

Prep Time: 15 minutes • Total Time: 45 minutes   Makes 4 servings

3   tablespoons coconut oil or organic butter, divided

1   large sweet onion, quartered and thinly sliced crosswise

8   shiitake or porcini mushrooms, sliced

1   bunch (12 ounces) organic spinach or chard, chopped

¼   teaspoon salt, divided

¼   teaspoon ground black pepper, divided

1   clove garlic, mashed with a mortar and pestle or in a mini food processor

6   eggs, lightly beaten

2   tablespoons chopped fresh parsley

2   tablespoons chopped fresh basil

2   teaspoons chopped fresh thyme

1. In a 10" skillet over low heat, heat 2 tablespoons of the oil or butter. Cook the onion, stirring occasionally, for 10 minutes, or until soft. Add the mushrooms and cook, stirring occasionally, for 5 minutes, or until soft. Add the spinach or chard and cook, stirring occasionally, for 5 minutes, or until all of the moisture has cooked off and the greens are tender. Season with ⅛ teaspoon of the salt and ⅛ teaspoon of the pepper. Transfer to a plate and set aside.

2. In a medium bowl, combine the garlic and the remaining ⅛ teaspoon salt. Add the eggs, parsley, basil, and thyme. Whisk well.

3. In the same skillet over medium heat, heat the remaining 1 tablespoon oil or butter. When the oil begins to sizzle or the butter begins to brown, swirl around the pan. Add the egg mixture, along with the remaining ⅛ teaspoon pepper. Cook for 1 to 2 minutes, pulling up the edges with a heatproof silicone spatula to allow the uncooked egg to flow underneath, or until the bottom is golden brown and the top begins to set but is still a bit moist.

4. Scatter the onion mixture over the center. Cook for 1 minute, or until heated through. Using the spatula, fold up one-third of the omelet. Roll the omelet over onto itself, tilt the pan, and slide the omelet onto a serving plate.

Per serving: 258 calories, 14 g protein, 13 g carbohydrates, 18 g total fat, 11 g saturated fat, 4 g fiber, 548 mg sodium

Quinoa Porridge

Prep Time: 5 minutes • Total Time: 35 minutes   Makes 2 servings

¼ cup macadamia nuts

1½ cups water

⅓ cup quinoa

1 teaspoon vanilla extract

Pinch of salt

1 cinnamon stick or pinch of cinnamon

Stevia to taste

1. In a high-powered blender or Vitamix, combine the macadamia nuts and water. Blend on high for 2 minutes to make nut milk.

2. In a small saucepan over medium-high heat, combine the nut milk and quinoa. Bring to a boil. Add the vanilla, salt, cinnamon, and stevia. Reduce the heat to low and simmer for 25 to 35 minutes, or until the quinoa is cooked and all of the liquid has been absorbed. Remove the cinnamon stick, if used, before serving.

Per serving: 229 calories, 5 g protein, 21 g carbohydrates, 14 g total fat, 2 g saturated fat, 3 g fiber, 82 mg sodium

Dandelion Greens with Hot Olive Oil Dressing

Prep Time: 10 minutes • Total Time: 15 minutes   Makes 4 servings

¼   cup extra-virgin olive oil

3   cloves garlic, thinly sliced lengthwise

⅓   cup sliced almonds

½   cup golden raisins

2   tablespoons sherry vinegar

¼   teaspoon salt

¼   teaspoon ground black pepper

1   bunch tender young dandelion greens, arugula, or baby spinach, chopped into bite-size pieces

1   bunch arugula or Bibb lettuce, chopped into bite-size pieces

1. In a 10" heavy skillet over medium-high heat, heat the oil for 1 minute, or until hot. Cook the garlic and almonds, stirring frequently, for 2 minutes, or until pale golden. Add the raisins and cook, stirring, for 1 minute, or until the raisins are plumped. Remove the pan from the heat and add the vinegar, salt, and pepper, stirring until combined. Set aside.

2. In a large serving bowl, combine the dandelion greens and lettuce. Pour the reserved hot dressing over the greens, tossing to coat.

Per serving: 259 calories, 4 g protein, 22 g carbohydrates, 18 g total fat, 2 g saturated fat, 3 g fiber, 180 mg sodium

Lentil Salad

Prep Time: 10 minutes • Total Time: 35 minutes   Makes 4 servings

- 1 cup uncooked red or brown lentils
- 1 red onion, chopped (1 cup)
- 1 red bell pepper, chopped (½ cup)
- ½ cup chopped fresh parsley or cilantro
- 2 tablespoons unfiltered apple cider vinegar
- 2 cloves garlic, crushed
- 2 tablespoons Dijon mustard
- 2–3 tablespoons fresh lemon juice
- 2 tablespoons chopped dill
- 1 cup broccoli sprouts, mung bean sprouts, or other sprouts

1. In a medium saucepan over medium-high heat, bring 2 cups of water to a boil. Simmer the lentils for 15 minutes, or until soft but still maintaining their shape. Drain, if necessary. Add the onion, pepper, and parsley or cilantro.

2. In a small bowl, whisk the vinegar, garlic, mustard, lemon juice, and dill until combined. Pour over the lentil mixture and mix well. Top with the sprouts. Serve warm or at room temperature.

Per serving: 217 calories, 15 g protein, 38 g carbohydrates, 1 g total fat, 0 g saturated fat, 9 g fiber, 195 mg sodium

Watercress Salad

Makes 6 servings

½ cup extra-virgin olive oil

¼ cup rice vinegar

2 tablespoons chopped fresh basil

2 tablespoons chopped fresh chives

1 tablespoon minced shallot

1 teaspoon Dijon mustard

1 clove garlic, minced

⅛ teaspoon salt

⅛ teaspoon ground black pepper

1 pound watercress, tough stems removed, chopped

1 large yellow tomato (when in season), cut into bite-size wedges

1 sweet onion, thinly sliced

1 large cucumber, quartered lengthwise and sliced

1 red bell pepper, cut into short strips

1 cup radishes, cut into bite-size pieces

1 avocado, cubed

1. In a container with a tightly sealed lid (such as a canning jar), combine the oil, vinegar, basil, chives, shallots, mustard, garlic, salt, and black pepper. Cover tightly and shake until the dressing is emulsified.

2. In a large bowl, toss the watercress, tomato, onion, cucumber, bell pepper, and radishes. Drizzle with the vinaigrette and toss to coat. Add the avocado just before serving.

TIP: *You can make the vinaigrette ahead of time. Simply cover and refrigerate it until you're ready to use it. Shake it well before drizzling it over the salad.*

Per serving: 256 calories, 4 g protein, 12 g carbohydrates, 23 g total fat, 3 g saturated fat, 4 g fiber, 125 mg sodium

Fennel Salad with Olives

Prep Time: 10 minutes • Total Time: 15 minutes Makes 4 servings

⅓   cup extra-virgin olive oil

2   tablespoons fresh lemon juice

2   small fennel bulbs, thinly sliced

1   large tart apple, cored and sliced

½   cup chopped black olives

Chopped parsley (optional)

1. In a small bowl, whisk together the oil and lemon juice.

2. In a large bowl, combine the fennel, apple, and olives. Add the dressing and toss to coat. Sprinkle with parsley, if desired.

Per serving: 255 calories, 2 g protein, 17 g carbohydrates, 21 g total fat, 3 g saturated fat, 5 g fiber, 186 mg sodium

Simple Summer Salad

Prep Time: 15 minutes • Total Time: 30 minutes   Makes 4 servings

8   ounces asparagus, chopped into 1"
     pieces

5   radishes, sliced

1   tablespoon white wine vinegar

3   tablespoons extra-virgin olive oil

¼   teaspoon salt

¼   teaspoon ground black pepper

1   small cucumber, sliced

1   cup red and yellow cherry tomatoes,
     halved

     Kernels from 2 ears raw sweet corn

1   avocado, chopped

1   cup baby arugula

1   shallot, minced

1   teaspoon chopped fresh basil

1   teaspoon chopped fresh oregano

1   teaspoon fresh lemon juice
     (optional)

1. In a tea kettle or saucepan, boil 3 cups of water. In a large bowl, combine the asparagus and radishes. Pour the boiling water over the vegetables. Allow to sit for 2 to 5 minutes, or until the vegetables are tender-crisp. Drain the water. Set aside. In a small bowl, whisk together the vinegar, oil, salt, and pepper.

2. In a large bowl, combine the reserved asparagus mixture and the remaining vegetables and herbs. Drizzle with the dressing and toss to coat. Sprinkle with lemon juice, if desired, just before serving.

Per serving: 229 calories, 5 g protein, 20 g carbohydrates, 17 g total fat, 3 g saturated fat, 5 g fiber, 162 mg sodium

Autumn Arugula Salad

Prep Time: 15 minutes • Total Time: 25 minutes

Makes 4 servings

⅓ cup walnuts, coarsely chopped

2 teaspoons grainy mustard

1 shallot, minced

3 tablespoons apple cider vinegar

3–5 drops stevia (to taste)

¼ cup extra-virgin olive oil

¼ teaspoon coarse salt

¼ teaspoon ground black pepper

2 Granny Smith or Gala apples (preferably organic), sliced paper thin

4 cups baby arugula

1 large head Belgian endive, leaves separated

2 tablespoons coarsely chopped fresh mint leaves

1. In a small skillet over medium heat, toast the walnuts, stirring frequently, for 5 minutes, or until crisp and fragrant. Remove from the heat and set aside.

2. In a large bowl, whisk the mustard, shallot, vinegar, and stevia until well combined. Whisk in the oil until thick; season with the salt and pepper.

3. Add the apples and arugula and toss to coat with the dressing. Arrange the endive leaves on 4 serving plates. Top with the apple mixture and scatter the mint and reserved walnuts over the top.

Per serving: 244 calories, 3 g protein, 17 g carbohydrates, 20 g total fat, 3 g saturated fat, 3 g fiber, 188 mg sodium

Kale and Brussels Sprouts Salad

Prep Time: 20 minutes • Total Time: 25 minutes   Makes 4 servings

2   large bunches Tuscan kale, center stems discarded and leaves thinly sliced (about 10 ounces after trimming)

12   ounces Brussels sprouts, trimmed and shredded

¼   cup fresh lemon juice

2   tablespoons Dijon mustard

1   tablespoon minced shallot

1   small clove garlic, finely grated

¼   teaspoon kosher salt

¼   teaspoon ground black pepper

½   cup extra-virgin olive oil

⅓   cup walnuts or almonds, toasted (optional)

1. In a large bowl, combine the kale and Brussels sprouts.

2. In a small bowl, combine the lemon juice, mustard, shallot, garlic, salt, and pepper. Whisk to blend. Slowly whisk in the oil until thick.

3. Pour the dressing over the kale mixture and toss to coat. Season to taste with additional pepper, if desired. Garnish with the nuts, if desired.

TIP: For busy nights, make the dressing ahead of time and store in the refrigerator until ready to use.

Per serving: 385 calories, 7 g protein, 18 g carbohydrates, 34 g total fat, 5 g saturated fat, 5 g fiber, 467 mg sodium

Cabbage and Daikon Salad with Sprouts

Prep Time: 15 minutes • Total Time: 20 minutes   Makes 6 servings

1 small green cabbage	3 tablespoons unrefined apple cider vinegar (such as Bragg's)
¼ head napa cabbage	2 teaspoons Dijon mustard
½ daikon or 10 red radishes	½ cup extra-virgin olive oil
2 ribs celery	3 tablespoons chopped fresh basil (optional)
1 small sweet onion	¼ teaspoon ground black pepper
2 cups broccoli sprouts, adzuki bean sprouts, chickpea sprouts, alfalfa sprouts, or mung bean sprouts (see Tip)	

1. Using a mandoline, the slicing blade of a food processor, or a sharp knife, slice the cabbages, daikon or radishes, celery, and onion very thinly. (You should have about 10 cups of green cabbage and 2 cups of napa or Chinese cabbage.) Toss together in a large bowl. Add the sprouts and toss to combine.

2. In a small bowl or a jar with a lid, combine the vinegar, mustard, oil, basil (if desired), and pepper. Whisk or shake until thick.

3. Add the dressing to the vegetables and toss to combine. Season to taste with additional pepper, if desired. The salad can be made ahead of time and will keep for a couple of days in the refrigerator.

TIP: *Napa cabbage is also known as Chinese cabbage. The sprouts can be purchased or grown at home. See the recipe on page 99.*

Per serving: 249 calories, 4 g protein, 18 g carbohydrates, 19 g total fat, 3 g saturated fat, 6 g fiber, 95 mg sodium

Arugula, Pomegranate, and Pecan Salad

Prep Time: 10 minutes • Total Time: 15 minutes   **Makes 4 servings**

1½   teaspoons red wine vinegar

1–2   tablespoons aged balsamic vinegar

¼   teaspoon salt

¼   teaspoon ground black pepper

6   tablespoons extra-virgin olive oil

2   medium bunches baby organic arugula (about 8 ounces)

⅓   cup pecans, toasted and roughly chopped

½   cup pomegranate seeds (from 1 medium pomegranate)

1. In a medium glass bowl, whisk together the vinegars, salt, and pepper. Gradually drizzle in the oil, whisking until thick.

2. In a large bowl, toss the arugula with just enough vinaigrette to coat. Divide the salad among 4 salad plates. Top each with the pecans and pomegranate seeds.

Per serving: 278 calories, 2 g protein, 7 g carbohydrates, 27 g total fat, 3 g saturated fat, 2 g fiber, 197 mg sodium

Bok Choy and Apple Salad

Prep Time: 10 minutes • Total Time: 15 minutes   Makes 2 servings

- 5 stalks bok choy (about ½ head), thinly sliced
- ½ small red onion, thinly sliced
- 1 Granny Smith apple (or any crunchy apple), sliced
- 2 tablespoons apple cider vinegar or fresh lemon juice
- ¼ cup extra-virgin olive oil
- 1 teaspoon ground coriander
- 1 teaspoon Dijon mustard
- ¼ teaspoon salt
- ¼ teaspoon ground black pepper

1. In a large bowl, combine the bok choy, onion, and apple. Toss well.

2. In a small bowl, combine the vinegar or lemon juice, oil, coriander, mustard, salt, and pepper. Whisk until thick. Drizzle over the salad and toss to coat. Serve immediately.

TIP: *This salad can be made ahead and then chilled for up to 1 hour. Add the apples just before serving.*

VARIATIONS: *Cabbage can be substituted for the bok choy, and scallions or carrot slices can be used instead of the onion. If desired, add fresh herbs such as cilantro, parsley, or mint. You can also double the dressing and use it on leftover cooked grains.*

Per serving: 322 calories, 4 g protein, 19 g carbohydrates, 29 g total fat, 4 g saturated fat, 4 g fiber, 489 mg sodium

Arugula and Pear Salad

Prep Time: 5 minutes • Total Time: 10 minutes   Makes 1 serving

5   ounces organic arugula or spinach (about 5 cups)

2   tablespoons extra-virgin olive oil

1   tablespoon fresh lemon juice

$\frac{1}{4}$ teaspoon grated lemon peel

1   pear, very thinly sliced

2   tablespoons pecans, toasted

$\frac{1}{4}$ teaspoon ground black pepper

1. In a salad bowl, toss the arugula or spinach with the oil, lemon juice, and lemon peel.

2. Top with the pear slices and sprinkle with the pecans. Season with the pepper.

Per serving: 479 calories, 6 g protein, 36 g carbohydrates, 38 g total fat, 5 g saturated fat, 9 g fiber, 40 mg sodium

Winter Bean Salad

Prep Time: 10 minutes • Total Time: 25 minutes   Makes 4 servings

¼ cup coconut oil

1 teaspoon ground cumin

1½ cups frozen edamame, thawed

1 can (15 ounces) black beans, rinsed and drained

1 can (15 ounces) black-eyed peas, rinsed and drained

¼ cup chopped red onion

2 cups thinly sliced organic celery

2 tablespoons fresh lime juice

½ cup chopped fresh cilantro

2 cloves garlic, chopped

¼ teaspoon salt

¼ teaspoon ground black pepper

1. In a small heavy saucepan or skillet over medium-low heat, heat the oil. Cook the cumin, stirring, for 30 seconds, or until fragrant and a bit darker. Pour into a heatproof bowl.

2. Add the edamame, black beans, peas, onion, celery, lime juice, cilantro, garlic, salt, and pepper. Toss to coat. Let stand for 10 minutes to allow the flavors to blend.

Per serving: 295 calories, 12 g protein, 27 g carbohydrates, 17 g total fat, 12 g saturated fat, 8 g fiber, 623 mg sodium

Adzuki Bean and Quinoa Salad with Cilantro Chile Dressing

Prep Time: 20 minutes + soaking time
Total Time: 1 hour 45 minutes + soaking time

Makes 6 servings

1½ cups dried adzuki beans or 3 cans (15 ounces each), rinsed and drained)

1½ cups quinoa

1–2 cloves garlic

1 jalapeño chile pepper, seeded if desired (wear plastic gloves when handling)

1 cup loosely packed fresh cilantro, rinsed and spun dry

¼ cup fresh lemon or lime juice

½ cup extra-virgin olive oil

¼ teaspoon salt

1 red bell pepper, chopped

1 bunch organic arugula (4 cups)

1. If using dried beans, in a medium bowl, cover the beans with water and soak overnight. Drain.

2. In a medium saucepan over medium heat, simmer the beans in 4 cups of water for 30 to 40 minutes, or until just tender but still holding their shape. Drain and allow to cool. Meanwhile, in a medium saucepan over medium heat, simmer the quinoa in 2½ cups of water for 15 to 20 minutes, or until the water is absorbed and the quinoa is fluffy.

3. In a blender, combine the garlic, jalapeño pepper, cilantro, lemon or lime juice, oil, and salt. Puree, scraping down the side of the blender as needed, until the dressing is smooth.

4. In a very large bowl, toss the beans, quinoa, and bell pepper with the dressing. Allow to marinate, covered and chilled, for at least 30 minutes before serving. Serve on a bed of arugula.

Per serving: 492 calories, 16 g protein, 61 g carbohydrates, 22 g total fat, 3 g saturated fat, 10 g fiber, 106 mg sodium

Quinoa and Toasted Vegetable Salad

Prep Time: 10 minutes • Total Time: 30 minutes　　　　　　Makes 6 servings

2　tablespoons extra-virgin olive oil

2　tablespoons fresh lemon juice

3　large cloves garlic, minced, divided

½　teaspoon finely grated lemon peel

2　tablespoons coconut oil, divided

1⅓　cups quinoa

½ teaspoon salt, divided

1¾　cups low-sodium vegetable broth + additional if needed

8–10 slender asparagus spears, trimmed, cut diagonally into ¾" pieces (about 2½ cups)

8　ounces sugar snap peas, trimmed, cut diagonally into ½" pieces (about 2½ cups)

1　cup shelled fresh green peas (or frozen if peas aren't in season)

¼　teaspoon ground black pepper

1　bunch arugula (4 ounces), chopped

⅓　cup chopped fresh chives

⅓　cup alfalfa sprouts

1. In a small bowl, whisk together the olive oil, lemon juice, two-thirds of the garlic, and the lemon peel. Set the dressing aside.

2. In a heavy medium saucepan over medium heat, heat 1 tablespoon of the coconut oil. Add the quinoa and ¼ teaspoon of the salt and cook, stirring frequently, for 5 minutes, or until most of the quinoa is golden brown. Add the broth, increase the heat to medium-high, and bring to a boil. Reduce the heat to medium-low, cover, and simmer for 10 minutes, or until the liquid is absorbed and the quinoa is fluffy. Add more broth if it becomes too dry.

3. Meanwhile, in a heavy large skillet over medium heat, heat the remaining 1 tablespoon coconut oil. Cook the asparagus, sugar snap peas, green peas, remaining garlic, remaining ¼ teaspoon salt, and pepper for 3 minutes, or until tender-crisp. Transfer to a large bowl.

4. Add the quinoa and arugula to the vegetables. Drizzle the reserved dressing over the salad. Add the chives and sprouts. Toss. Season with additional salt and pepper, if desired.

Per serving: 303 calories, 10 g protein, 36 g carbohydrates, 14 g total fat, 7 g saturated fat, 7 g fiber, 289 mg sodium

Kale, Squash, and White Bean Salad

Prep Time: 20 minutes • Total Time: 45 minutes

Makes 4 servings

- 2 medium delicata squashes or 1 medium peeled butternut squash (about 2 pounds), halved lengthwise and seeded
- 3 tablespoons coconut oil, divided
- 2 tablespoons balsamic vinegar, divided
- ½ bunch kale (5 ounces), large stems removed, cut into 1" pieces
- 1 large shallot, finely chopped
- 1 clove garlic, minced
- 1 tablespoon red wine vinegar
- 1 teaspoon coarse salt
- ¼ teaspoon ground black pepper
- 1 can (15 ounces) cannellini beans, rinsed and drained

1. Preheat the oven to 400°F. Line a baking sheet with parchment paper.

2. If using delicata squash, cut into ½"-thick semicircles. If using butternut squash, cut into cubes. In a large bowl, toss the squash with 1½ tablespoons of the oil. Spread onto the baking sheet and bake for 15 to 18 minutes, or until just tender. Brush 1 tablespoon of the balsamic vinegar onto the squash. Bake for 5 minutes.

3. Meanwhile, place the kale in a large bowl. In a small saucepan over medium heat, heat the remaining 1½ tablespoons oil. Cook the shallot and garlic for 4 minutes, or until slightly softened. Add the red wine vinegar and remaining 1 tablespoon balsamic vinegar and bring to a boil. Immediately pour the hot dressing over the kale. Sprinkle with the salt and season with the pepper.

4. Add the squash and beans. Cover and let stand for 5 minutes. Toss until the kale wilts slightly. Serve warm or at room temperature.

Per serving: 300 calories, 9 g protein, 48 g carbohydrates, 11 g total fat, 9 g saturated fat, 9 g fiber, 686 mg sodium

Yummy Black Bean Burgers

Prep Time: 10 minutes • Total Time: 1 hour   Makes 6

½   cup quinoa

½   teaspoon salt

1   small onion or 2 shallots, finely chopped

6   sun-dried tomatoes packed in olive oil, finely chopped (about ¼ cup)

2   cans (15 ounces each) black beans, rinsed and drained, or 2½ cups cooked

2   large cloves garlic, minced

1   teaspoon chili powder

½   teaspoon ground cumin

¼   teaspoon ground black pepper

1. In a small saucepan over medium-high heat, combine the quinoa, ¾ cup of water, and the salt. Bring to a boil. Cover, reduce the heat to medium-low, and simmer for 10 to 15 minutes, or until all of the liquid is absorbed.

2. Meanwhile, in a medium skillet over medium-low heat, cook the onion or shallots and the tomatoes for 3 to 4 minutes, or until the onion has softened. (The oil left on the tomatoes should be enough to cook the onion.) Stir in 1¼ cups of the black beans, the garlic, chili powder, cumin, and 1 cup of water. Simmer for 9 to 11 minutes, or until most of the liquid has evaporated. (The mixture should have the consistency of refried beans.)

3. Transfer the bean mixture to a food processor, add half of the cooked quinoa, and process until smooth. Transfer to a bowl and stir in the remaining quinoa and remaining 1¼ cups black beans. Season with the black pepper and additional salt, if desired. Allow mixture to cool.

4. Preheat the oven to 350°F and generously coat a baking sheet with coconut oil or butter. Shape the bean mixture into 6 patties and place on the baking sheet. Bake for 20 minutes, or until the patties are crisp on top. Turn the patties with a spatula and bake for 10 minutes, or until both sides are crisp and brown.

Per serving (1 burger): 142 calories, 7 g protein, 26 g carbohydrates, 2 g total fat, 0 g saturated fat, 6 g fiber, 534 mg sodium

Salmon Avocado Wraps

Prep Time: 5 minutes • Total Time: 10 minutes   Makes 4

1   can (6 ounces) wild-caught Alaskan salmon

½   cup chopped scallions

2   tablespoons chopped fresh parsley

1   tablespoon extra-virgin olive oil

1   tablespoon fresh lime juice

½   cup broccoli sprouts, adzuki bean sprouts, chickpea sprouts, alfalfa sprouts, or mung bean sprouts (see Tip)

¼   teaspoon salt

¼   teaspoon ground black pepper

4   large bok choy or Chinese cabbage leaves

¼   cup chopped avocado

½   cup cherry tomatoes, halved

In a large mixing bowl, combine the salmon, scallions, parsley, oil, lime juice, sprouts, salt, and pepper. Divide the mixture among the bok choy or Chinese cabbage leaves. Top with the avocado and tomatoes and fold into wraps.

TIP: *See the recipe for growing your own sprouts on page 99, or purchase them at a health food store.*

Per serving (2 wraps): 242 calories, 19 g protein, 7 g carbohydrates, 16 g total fat, 3 g saturated fat, 3 g fiber, 617 mg sodium

Curried Quinoa and Chickpea Lettuce Wraps

Prep Time: 15 minutes • Total Time: 45 minutes   Makes 8

1 tablespoon Madras curry powder	⅓ cup olive oil
1½ cups water	¼ cup white wine vinegar
¼ teaspoon salt	1 tablespoon grated fresh ginger (or more to taste)
4 cups fresh vegetables (such as a mixture of broccoli florets, cauliflower florets, and thinly sliced carrots)	1 cup thinly sliced scallions
	2 cups broccoli sprouts, alfalfa sprouts, chickpea sprouts, adzuki sprouts, lentil sprouts, or mung bean sprouts
1 cup quinoa	
1 can (15 ounces) chickpeas, rinsed and drained	8 large romaine lettuce or Swiss chard leaves

1. In a heavy, large saucepan over medium-high heat, cook the curry powder for 1 minute, or until fragrant and toasted. Mix in the water and salt. Bring to a boil. Plunge the vegetables in the boiling water for 1 minute to blanch. With a slotted spoon, transfer the vegetables to a bowl and set aside.

2. Bring the water in the saucepan back to a boil. Add the quinoa and stir. Reduce the heat to medium-low, cover, and cook for 20 minutes, or until the water is absorbed and the quinoa is fluffy. Do not overcook.

3. Add the quinoa to the reserved vegetables. Add the chickpeas, oil, vinegar, and ginger. Allow to cool to room temperature. Add the scallions and sprouts. Toss. Season to taste with additional salt, if needed.

4. Spoon a small dollop of the mixture in the center of a lettuce leaf. Roll the bottom edge over the mixture. Tuck in the sides. Roll up to the top edge. Repeat for the remaining vegetable mixture and lettuce leaves.

Per serving (2 wraps): 432 calories, 12 g protein, 45 g carbohydrates, 23 g total fat, 3 g saturated fat, 10 g fiber, 371 mg sodium

Avocado Egg Salad Wraps

Prep Time: 5 minutes • Total Time: 10 minutes   Makes 4

3 hard-cooked eggs	¼ teaspoon Dijon mustard
1 medium avocado, halved, pitted, peeled, and mashed	⅛ teaspoon salt
1 tablespoon extra-virgin olive oil	⅛ teaspoon ground black pepper
1 tablespoon fresh lemon juice	1 tablespoon chopped fresh basil (optional)
1 tablespoon chopped scallions	4 large romaine lettuce or Swiss chard leaves

1. In a medium bowl, combine the eggs, avocado, oil, lemon juice, scallions, and mustard. Mash with a fork. Add the salt, pepper, and basil (if desired) and stir to combine.

2. Spoon one-quarter of the mixture in the center of a lettuce leaf. Roll the bottom edge over the mixture. Tuck in the sides. Roll up to the top edge. Repeat for the remaining egg mixture and lettuce leaves.

TIP: *Because avocados turn brown quickly, this egg salad is best served on the day it's made.*

Per serving (2 wraps): 307 calories, 12 g protein, 10 g carbohydrates, 25 g total fat, 5 g saturated fat, 6 g fiber, 260 mg sodium

Moroccan Quinoa

Prep Time: 5 minutes • Total Time: 30 minutes   Makes 6 servings

1   cup quinoa

1   tablespoon coconut oil

1   small onion, finely chopped

1   teaspoon ground cumin

½   teaspoon ground cinnamon

¼   teaspoon ground turmeric

1   cup low-sodium vegetable broth

⅔   cup water

⅓   cup dried currants or raisins

½   teaspoon salt

3   tablespoons finely chopped fresh parsley or cilantro leaves

¼   cup mung bean sprouts

1. In a fine strainer, rinse the quinoa under cold running water until the water is clear. Drain well. Set aside.

2. In a heavy saucepan over medium-low heat, heat the oil. Cook the onion, stirring frequently, for 4 minutes, or until softened. Add the cumin, cinnamon, and turmeric. Cook, stirring, for 30 seconds.

3. Add the reserved quinoa and cook, stirring, for 1 minute. Add the broth, water, currants or raisins, and salt. Increase the heat to medium-high and bring to a boil. Reduce the heat to medium-low and simmer, covered, for 15 minutes, or until the liquid is absorbed.

4. Remove the pan from the heat. Allow the mixture to stand, covered, for 5 minutes. Stir in the parsley or cilantro and the sprouts.

Per serving: 158 calories, 5 g protein, 26 g carbohydrates, 4 g total fat, 2 g saturated fat, 3 g fiber, 222 mg sodium

Quinoa with Lemon and Pine Nuts

Prep Time: 10 minutes • Total Time: 40 minutes   Makes 4 servings

1 cup quinoa	⅓ cup pine nuts, lightly toasted
1½ cups water	½ cup finely chopped red onion
¼ teaspoon salt	⅛ teaspoon ground black pepper
1 tablespoon extra-virgin olive oil	½ cup chopped fresh basil
1½ teaspoons fresh lemon juice	

1. In a fine strainer, rinse the quinoa under cold running water until the water is clear.

2. In a medium saucepan over medium-high heat, combine the quinoa, water, and salt. Bring to a boil. Reduce the heat to medium-low, cover, and simmer for 15 minutes, or until the water is absorbed and the quinoa is tender. Do not overcook. Transfer the quinoa to a large serving bowl. Fluff with a fork.

3. In a small bowl, combine the oil and lemon juice. Stir into the quinoa. Cool to room temperature. Add the pine nuts and onion and stir to combine. Season with additional salt, the pepper, and basil. Stir to combine.

TIP: *This dish can be prepared up to 6 hours ahead. Cover and chill in the refrigerator.*

Per serving: 273 calories, 8 g protein, 31 g carbohydrates, 14 g total fat, 1 g saturated fat, 4 g fiber, 225 mg sodium

Ginger Miso Sweet Potatoes with Sautéed Greens

Prep Time: 15 minutes • Total Time: 1 hour 5 minutes   **Makes 4 servings**

2   small sweet potatoes or yams (1 pound)

2   tablespoons white miso paste

1   tablespoon smooth, organic peanut butter

1   tablespoon coconut oil

2   tablespoons finely chopped shallot

1   tablespoon finely chopped fresh ginger

2   cloves garlic, minced

8   collard green, kale, or chard leaves, stems removed, finely chopped

1   cup frozen shelled edamame

2   tablespoons water

1/4 teaspoon ground red pepper

2   tablespoons chopped fresh cilantro

1. Preheat the oven to 400°F. Cut a thin slice off both ends of the sweet potatoes or yams and poke the skins with a knife in several places. Bake for 50 minutes, turning once, or until soft. Slice in half and scoop the flesh into a bowl. Add the miso and peanut butter and mash until combined.

2. Meanwhile, in a medium skillet over medium heat, melt the oil. Cook the shallot, ginger, and garlic for 3 minutes, or until soft. Add the greens, edamame, water, and pepper and cook for 3 minutes, or until the greens are wilted. Transfer to the sweet potato mixture. Add the cilantro and stir until combined. Serve warm or at room temperature. This dish is delicious the next day.

Per serving: 148 calories, 6 g protein, 16 g carbohydrates, 7 g total fat, 3 g saturated fat, 4 g fiber, 270 mg sodium

Hearty Cleansing Soup

Prep Time: 20 minutes • Total Time: 1 hour   Makes 12 servings

- 2 teaspoons coconut oil
- 1 pound organic, free-range ground beef, ground turkey, or shredded chicken
- 1 onion, chopped
- 2 cloves garlic, chopped
- 8 ounces mushrooms, chopped
- 2 quarts organic chicken or vegetable broth
- 1 can (15 ounces) organic crushed tomatoes
- 1 can (28 ounces) organic diced tomatoes

- 1 tablespoon fresh lemon juice (optional)
- 1 can (15 ounces) navy beans, rinsed and drained
- 2 teaspoons ground cumin
- 1/8 teaspoon crushed red-pepper flakes, or to taste
- 2 cups chopped kale leaves
- 1/4 cup fresh cilantro, chopped
- 1/4 cup fresh parsley, chopped

1. In a large pot over medium-high heat, heat the oil. Cook the beef or poultry for 5 minutes, stirring frequently, or until no longer pink. Drain and transfer to a plate. Set aside.

2. In the same pot, cook the onion, garlic, and mushrooms for 5 minutes, or until soft. Add the broth, crushed and diced tomatoes, lemon juice (if desired), beans, cumin, pepper flakes, kale, and reserved beef or poultry. Stir to combine. Cover and simmer for 20 minutes. Uncover and simmer for 10 minutes. Add the cilantro and parsley and stir to combine.

TIP: *This soup will keep in the refrigerator up to 5 days. It also freezes well.*

Per serving: 129 calories, 12 g protein, 12 g carbohydrates, 3 g total fat, 2 g saturated fat, 3 g fiber, 529 mg sodium

Watercress Soup

Prep Time: 10 minutes • Total Time: 40 minutes   Makes 4 servings

1 tablespoon coconut oil	6 cups low-sodium vegetable or chicken broth
1 large onion, quartered	
1 cup celery leaves	½ teaspoon sea salt, or to taste
8 large cloves garlic	1 bunch watercress, washed, large stems removed, chopped

1. In a large pot over medium heat, heat the oil. Cook the onion for 5 minutes, stirring frequently, or until translucent. Add the celery leaves and garlic and cook for 5 minutes. Add the broth and salt. Simmer for 10 minutes.

2. Transfer to a blender or food processor. Blend or process until very smooth. Return to the pot and season with additional salt, if desired. Add the watercress and bring to a boil. Stir and remove the pot from the heat. Allow to sit for a few minutes before serving.

Per serving: 57 calories, 1 g protein, 6 g carbohydrates, 4 g total fat, 3 g saturated fat, 1 g fiber, 221 mg sodium

Broccoli and Fennel Soup

Prep Time: 10 minutes • Total Time: 45 minutes   Makes 4 servings

1   tablespoon coconut oil

1   large onion, quartered

6   cloves garlic, sliced

1   large head broccoli, separated into florets and stems (woody stem portion removed)

1   small bulb fennel, chopped

6   cups low-sodium vegetable broth or water

½   teaspoon salt

¼   teaspoon ground black pepper

Feathery tops from fennel bulb for garnish

1. In a large pot over medium heat, heat the oil. Cook the onion and garlic for 5 minutes, stirring frequently, or until the onion is translucent. Add the broccoli and fennel and cook for 10 minutes, or until tender-crisp. Add the broth or water. Simmer for 10 to 15 minutes, or until the vegetables are tender.

2. Working in batches if necessary, transfer to a blender or food processor. Blend or process until very smooth. Return to the pot, add the salt and pepper, and simmer for 10 minutes, or until heated through. Serve garnished with fennel tops.

Per serving: 122 calories, 6 g protein, 19 g carbohydrates, 4 g total fat, 3 g saturated fat, 7 g fiber, 374 mg sodium

Gazpacho

Prep Time: 20 minutes • Total Time: 25 minutes + chilling time **Makes 6 servings**

4   medium tomatoes, seeded and chopped, juices reserved

2   cloves garlic, chopped

2   cucumbers, peeled, seeded, and chopped

2   ribs celery, chopped

1   small onion, chopped, or 3 scallions, chopped

1   red bell pepper, cored, seeded, and chopped

1½   cups tomato or V8 juice

¼   cup balsamic or red wine vinegar

½   cup extra-virgin olive oil

¼   teaspoon ground red pepper

¼   teaspoon salt

¼   teaspoon ground black pepper

Chopped cilantro for garnish

1. In a large bowl, combine the tomatoes (with their juice), garlic, cucumbers, celery, onion or scallions, bell pepper, tomato or V8 juice, vinegar, oil, red pepper, salt, and black pepper. Transfer 2 cups of the mixture to another bowl.

2. Working in batches, transfer the remaining mixture to a blender or food processor. Pulse until just slightly chunky. Return to the bowl and add the reserved vegetable mixture and additional salt, if desired. Stir to combine. Serve chilled, garnished with chopped cilantro.

Per serving: 228 calories, 3 g protein, 13 g carbohydrates, 19 g total fat, 3 g saturated fat, 3 g fiber, 288 mg sodium

Tomato Curry Soup

Prep Time: 15 minutes • Total Time: 30 minutes   Makes 4 servings

2 tablespoons coconut oil	1/2 teaspoon ground cumin
1 small onion, chopped	1 bay leaf
2 cloves garlic, chopped	3 cups low-sodium vegetable or chicken broth
1 tablespoon finely chopped fresh ginger	
2 large tomatoes, chopped	1/4 teaspoon salt
1/2 teaspoon curry powder	1/4 teaspoon ground black pepper
	2 tablespoons chopped fresh cilantro

1. In a large pot over medium heat, heat the oil. Cook the onion, garlic, and ginger for 5 minutes, or until the onion is soft.

2. Add the tomatoes, curry powder, cumin, and bay leaf and stir to combine. Simmer for 5 minutes. Add the broth, salt, and pepper and simmer for 3 minutes, or until the soup is heated through. Remove from the heat and discard the bay leaf. Add the cilantro and stir to combine.

Per serving: 102 calories, 1 g protein, 8 g carbohydrates, 7 g total fat, 6 g saturated fat, 2 g fiber, 257 mg sodium

Artichoke Soup

Prep Time: 10 minutes • Total Time: 45 minutes   Makes 4 servings

2   tablespoons coconut oil

1   onion, chopped

8   cloves garlic, crushed

2   cans (14 ounces each) artichokes packed in water, rinsed, drained, and chopped

2   cups organic chicken or vegetable stock

2   teaspoons chopped fresh basil or 1 teaspoon dried

2   teaspoons chopped fresh oregano or 1 teaspoon dried

$\frac{1}{4}$ teaspoon salt

$\frac{1}{4}$ teaspoon ground red pepper

1. In a pot over medium-high heat, heat the oil. Cook the onion and garlic for 5 minutes, or until the onion is translucent.

2. Add the artichokes, stock, basil, oregano, salt, and pepper and stir to combine. Cover and simmer for 30 minutes, or until the flavors meld. If a creamier consistency is desired, transfer the soup (in batches if necessary) to a blender or food processor. Blend or process until smooth.

Per serving: 142 calories, 5 g protein, 17 g carbohydrates, 7 g total fat, 6 g saturated fat, 3 g fiber, 836 mg sodium

Curry Squash Soup with Coconut Milk

Prep Time: 15 minutes • Total Time: 1 hour   Makes 6 servings

- 2   tablespoons coconut oil
- 2   onions, finely chopped
- 3   cloves garlic, minced
- 1   tablespoon minced fresh ginger
- 1   tablespoon curry powder or paste
- 4   cups water or low-sodium chicken or vegetable broth
- 7–8 cups peeled and cubed butternut squash (1 three-pound squash)

- 2   teaspoons sugar
- ½   teaspoon salt
- ¼   teaspoon ground black pepper
- 1   can (14 ounces) unsweetened coconut milk
- 2   tablespoons fresh lemon juice (optional)

1. In a large pot over medium heat, heat the oil. Cook the onions, garlic, and ginger for 5 minutes, or until the onions are translucent. Add the curry and cook for 1 minute, tossing continuously.

2. Add the water or broth and bring to a boil. Add the squash, sugar, salt, and pepper and reduce the heat to a strong simmer. Simmer for 30 minutes, or until the squash is very tender. Add the coconut milk, stir, and simmer for 5 minutes. Stir in the lemon juice, if desired.

3. Working in batches, transfer the soup to a blender or food processor. Blend or process until smooth. Return to the pot and reheat before serving.

Per serving: 276 calories, 5 g protein, 28 g carbohydrates, 17 g total fat, 16 g saturated fat, 5 g fiber, 258 mg sodium

Simply Divine Pureed Cauliflower Soup

Prep Time: 10 minutes • Total Time: 45 minutes   Makes 8 servings

<table>
<tr><td>2</td><td>heads cauliflower, cut into large florets</td><td>½</td><td>teaspoon salt</td></tr>
<tr><td>2</td><td>quarts organic chicken or vegetable broth</td><td>½</td><td>teaspoon ground black pepper</td></tr>
<tr><td>4–6</td><td>cloves garlic, chopped</td><td></td><td>Ground nutmeg or ground red pepper</td></tr>
<tr><td>1</td><td>large sweet onion, quartered</td><td></td><td>Truffle oil or extra-virgin olive oil (optional)</td></tr>
<tr><td>2</td><td>teaspoons chopped fresh rosemary, dill, or tarragon</td><td></td><td></td></tr>
</table>

1. In a large pot over medium-high heat, combine the cauliflower and broth and bring to a boil. Add the garlic, onion, and herb and stir to combine. Reduce the heat to a simmer and cook for 20 minutes, or until the cauliflower is tender.

2. Working in batches, transfer the soup to a blender or food processor. Blend or process until smooth. Return to the pot, add the salt and black pepper, and reheat slowly. Add the nutmeg or red pepper to taste. Drizzle with truffle oil or olive oil just before serving, if desired.

Per serving: 63 calories, 4 g protein, 12 g carbohydrates, 0.5 g total fat, 0 g saturated fat, 3 g fiber, 763 mg sodium

Nannie's Healing Chicken Soup

Prep Time: 20 minutes • Total Time: 55 minutes   Makes 4 servings

- 4 tablespoons coconut oil
- 1 onion, chopped
- 2 carrots, chopped
- 2 ribs celery, chopped
- 2 bay leaves
- 1½ teaspoons chopped fresh thyme or ½ teaspoon dried
- 4 fresh sage leaves or ½ teaspoon dried

- 4 cloves garlic, chopped
- 2 quarts organic, free-range, low-sodium chicken broth
- 1 pound boneless, skinless, free-range chicken breasts or thighs, sliced into bite-size pieces
- ½ teaspoon salt
- ¼ teaspoon ground black pepper
- 1 bunch kale, finely chopped (about 5 cups)

1. In a pot over medium heat, heat the oil. Cook the onion, carrots, celery, bay leaves, thyme, and sage for 8 minutes, stirring occasionally, or until the onion softens and becomes translucent. Add the garlic and cook for 2 minutes.

2. Add the broth, increase the heat to high, and bring to a boil. Reduce the heat to low, cover the pot, and simmer for 10 minutes, or until the carrots soften. Add the chicken and simmer for 8 minutes, or until the chicken is cooked through. Season with the salt and pepper. Add the kale and heat until the kale is soft, but still bright green. Remove the bay leaves before serving.

Per serving: 350 calories, 33 g protein, 17 g carbohydrates, 17 g total fat, 13 g saturated fat, 3 g fiber, 634 mg sodium

Sauerkraut

Prep Time: 20 minutes • Total Time: 1 hour   Makes 6 servings

1 tablespoon coconut oil	½ cup apple cider
1 small onion, thinly sliced	½ cup water, or to taste
1 medium green cabbage, finely shredded	1 tablespoon sea or kosher salt
1¼ cups unfiltered apple cider vinegar with the "mother" (such as Bragg's)	1 teaspoon caraway seeds (optional)

1. In a saucepan over medium-high heat, heat the oil. Cook the onion, stirring constantly, until it begins to soften and turn translucent, being careful not to let it brown.

2. Add the cabbage, vinegar, cider, water, salt, and caraway seeds (if desired) and bring to a boil. Cover, reduce the heat, and simmer for 30 to 45 minutes, or until the cabbage is tender. If the cabbage gets too dry, add additional water.

TIP: *If you prefer your sauerkraut tangy, use less water. The sauerkraut will keep, refrigerated, for 2 weeks.*

Per serving: 97 calories, 2 g protein, 19 g carbohydrates, 3 g total fat, 2 g saturated fat, 4 g fiber, 1,209 mg sodium

Kimchi

Prep Time: 15 minutes
Total Time: 3 hours 20 minutes + chilling time

Makes 8 servings

2 pounds napa cabbage	2 teaspoons minced fresh ginger
1 tablespoon salt	$\frac{1}{2}$ cup less-sodium soy sauce
2 scallions, chopped	$\frac{1}{2}$ cup white vinegar
4 cloves garlic, minced	1–2 teaspoons sugar
1 tablespoon crushed red-pepper flakes, or to taste	Sesame oil (optional)

1. Chop the cabbage coarsely and place in a large bowl. Sprinkle with the salt and let stand at room temperature for 3 to 4 hours.

2. Using your hands, squeeze the cabbage dry and place in another bowl. Add the scallions, garlic, pepper flakes, ginger, soy sauce, vinegar, and sugar. Mix well. Refrigerate for at least 24 hours before serving. If desired, sprinkle a few drops of sesame oil on each serving.

TIP: *Napa cabbage is also known as Chinese cabbage.*

Per serving: 35 calories, 2 g protein, 6 g carbohydrates, 0 g total fat, 0 g saturated fat, 2 g fiber, 1,270 mg sodium

Roasted Cauliflower and Brussels Sprouts with Caramelized Onions and Garlic

Prep Time: 10 minutes • Total Time: 50 minutes   Makes 6 servings

- 3 tablespoons coconut oil, divided
- 2 large sweet onions, sliced into ¼" wedges
- ⅛ teaspoon coarse salt
- ⅛ teaspoon ground black pepper
- 1–2 tablespoons sliced garlic
- 1 head cauliflower, cut into florets
- 8 cups organic Brussels sprouts, trimmed and halved

1. Preheat the oven to 350°F. Put 1 tablespoon of the oil in a roasting pan. Place the pan in the preheating oven for 1 minute, or until the oil melts. Remove the pan from the oven.

2. In the roasting pan, toss the onions in the oil. Season with the salt and pepper. Roast for 15 to 20 minutes, or until the onions are translucent. Remove the pan from the oven.

3. Add the remaining 2 tablespoons of oil. (The oil will melt immediately.) Toss the garlic, cauliflower, and Brussels sprouts in the oil and season with additional salt and pepper, if desired. Roast for 25 to 30 minutes, tossing occasionally, or until the vegetables are tender and caramelized. If the garlic begins to get too dark, remove it and set aside while the other vegetables are roasting.

Per serving: 145 calories, 5 g protein, 19 g carbohydrates, 7 g total fat, 6 g saturated fat, 5 g fiber, 102 mg sodium

Roasted Cauliflower, Broccolini, and Chickpeas

Prep Time: 15 minutes • Total Time: 50 minutes   Makes 4 servings

3 tablespoons coconut oil

3 cups cauliflower florets
   (about 8 ounces)

3 cups coarsely chopped broccolini
   (about 8 ounces)

6–8 cloves garlic, coarsely chopped

1 can (15 ounces) chickpeas, rinsed
   and drained

1/2 teaspoon crushed red pepper

1/4 teaspoon salt

3 tablespoons chopped fresh parsley
   or basil

1. Preheat the oven to 450°F. Put the oil on a rimmed baking sheet or in a roasting pan and place in the preheating oven for 1 minute, or until the oil melts. Remove from the oven.

2. On the baking sheet, toss the cauliflower, broccolini, garlic, and chickpeas with the oil. Sprinkle with the red pepper and salt. Toss again to coat thoroughly. Bake for 22 minutes, stirring once, or until the vegetables are browned and tender-crisp. Sprinkle with the parsley or basil before serving.

Per serving: 197 calories, 7 g protein, 19 g carbohydrates, 12 g total fat, 9 g saturated fat, 5 g fiber, 342 mg sodium

Roasted Brussels Sprouts with Caramelized Onions

Prep Time: 10 minutes • Total Time: 1 hour

Makes 6 servings

3 tablespoons coconut oil, divided

1 large sweet onion, sliced into ¼" wedges

¼ teaspoon coarse salt

¼ teaspoon ground black pepper

8 cups organic Brussels sprouts, trimmed and halved

1. Preheat the oven to 350°F. Put 1 tablespoon of the oil in a roasting pan. Place the pan in the preheating oven for 1 minute, or until the oil melts. Remove the pan from the oven.

2. In the pan, toss the onion with the oil. Season with the salt and pepper. Roast for 15 minutes, or until translucent. Remove the pan from the oven.

3. Add the remaining 2 tablespoons oil. (The oil will melt immediately.) Toss the Brussels sprouts with the oil and onion and season with additional salt and pepper, if desired. Roast for 25 to 30 minutes, tossing occasionally, or until the vegetables are tender and caramelized.

Per serving: 121 calories, 4 g protein, 13 g carbohydrates, 7 g total fat, 6 g saturated fat, 5 g fiber, 96 mg sodium

Stir-Fried Cabbage and Edamame

Prep Time: 15 minutes • Total Time: 30 minutes   Makes 4 servings

1½ tablespoons coconut oil

    Pinch of hing (optional, for
    digestion)

½ teaspoon cumin seeds

1 green chile pepper, seeded and
   chopped

¼ teaspoon ground turmeric

½ cup shelled edamame

8 ounces cabbage, cut into ½" strips

¼ teaspoon salt

¼ teaspoon garam masala

2 tablespoons chopped cilantro leaves

1. In a skillet over medium-high heat, heat the oil for 30 seconds. Cook the hing (if desired), cumin seeds, chile pepper, and turmeric for 30 seconds, or until fragrant. Add the edamame and cook for 30 seconds, coating the edamame with the spices.

2. Reduce the heat to medium and add the cabbage and salt. Cook, stirring frequently, for 10 minutes, or until the cabbage is soft. Add the garam masala and cilantro. Serve hot.

TIP: *This recipe was inspired by an Indian dish called patta gobhi matar.*

Per serving: 109 calories, 4 g protein, 11 g carbohydrates, 6 g total fat, 5 g saturated fat, 5 g fiber, 178 mg sodium

Kale Slaw with Red Cabbage and Carrots

Prep Time: 10 minutes • Total Time: 15 minutes

Makes 4 servings

- 1 tablespoon extra-virgin olive oil
- 1 tablespoon Dijon mustard
- 1 teaspoon apple cider vinegar
- ⅛ teaspoon coarse salt
- ⅛ teaspoon ground black pepper
- 1½ cups kale leaves, cut into thin strips
- 1½ cups shredded red cabbage

- 1 carrot, cut into matchsticks
- ¼ cup fresh parsley leaves
- 2 tablespoons chopped red onion
- 2 tablespoons shelled unsalted sunflower seeds
- 2 tablespoons shelled unsalted pumpkin seeds
- 2 tablespoons hemp seeds

1. In a small bowl, whisk together the oil, mustard, and vinegar. Season with the salt and pepper.

2. In a large bowl, combine the kale, cabbage, carrot, parsley, and onion. Add the sunflower, pumpkin, and hemp seeds and stir to combine. Season with additional salt and pepper, if desired. Drizzle with the dressing and toss to coat.

Per serving: 138 calories, 5 g protein, 9 g carbohydrates, 10 g total fat, 1 g saturated fat, 2 g fiber, 191 mg sodium

Simple Curried Chickpeas and Kale

Prep Time: 10 minutes • Total Time: 30 minutes   Makes 2 servings

2   cups organic kale leaves

1   tablespoon coconut oil

2   cloves garlic, minced

1   can (15 ounces) organic chickpeas, rinsed and drained

1/2   teaspoon ground cumin

1/4   teaspoon ground coriander

1 1/2   teaspoons finely chopped fresh ginger or 1/8 teaspoon ground ginger

1/8   teaspoon salt

1/8–1/4   teaspoon garam masala

Ground red pepper to taste

1. Place the kale in a steamer basket fitted over a pot containing a few inches of water. Cover and bring the water to a boil. Steam the kale for 3 to 5 minutes, or until it's bright green and softened. Transfer to a cutting board and chop finely. Arrange on a serving dish.

2. In a medium skillet over low heat, heat the oil. Cook the garlic for 3 minutes, or until soft and light golden. Add the chickpeas and stir to coat with the oil and garlic. If the mixture is dry, add 1 tablespoon of water. Add the cumin, coriander, ginger, and salt and stir to combine. Cook, stirring frequently, for 5 minutes, or until the chickpeas are warmed through. Remove from the heat.

3. Add the garam masala and red pepper. Top the kale with the chickpea mixture. Serve hot or at room temperature.

TIP: *Garam masala is an Indian spice that can be found in the spices or ethnic foods section of most grocery stores. This dish is also delicious served the next day.*

Per serving: 222 calories, 10 g protein, 26 g carbohydrates, 10 g total fat, 6 g saturated fat, 8 g fiber, 557 mg sodium

Asparagus with Toasted Pine Nuts and Lemon Peel

Prep Time: 10 minutes • Total Time: 20 minutes   **Makes 4 servings**

3 tablespoons pine nuts

2 tablespoons coconut oil

2 bunches asparagus (about 30 spears), trimmed and cut into bite-size pieces

¼ teaspoon salt

¼ teaspoon ground black pepper

1 teaspoon lemon peel

1. In a large, dry skillet over medium-low heat, toast the pine nuts for 4 to 5 minutes, tossing frequently, or until golden. Transfer to a plate and set aside.

2. In the same skillet over medium heat, heat the oil. Cook the asparagus, salt, and pepper for 3 to 5 minutes, tossing occasionally, or until tender-crisp. Add the reserved pine nuts and toss to combine. Add the lemon peel and additional salt and pepper, if desired, and toss.

Per serving: 126 calories, 4 g protein, 6 g carbohydrates, 11 g total fat, 6 g saturated fat, 2 g fiber, 148 mg sodium

Asparagus with Dijon Sauce

Prep Time: 5 minutes • Total Time: 15 minutes   Makes 2 servings

1   bunch asparagus (about 15 spears), trimmed

1   teaspoon coconut oil, melted

1½ tablespoons Dijon mustard

2   tablespoons vegetable broth

¼   teaspoon salt

¼   teaspoon ground black pepper

½   teaspoon nutritional yeast (optional)

1. Preheat the oven to 425°F. On a baking sheet, toss the asparagus with the oil. Roast for 8 minutes, or until the asparagus is bright green and tender-crisp. Be careful not to overcook.

2. Meanwhile, in a small bowl, whisk the mustard with 1 tablespoon of the broth at a time. It should be the consistency of a sauce—not as thick as mustard but not as runny as broth. Drizzle the sauce over the asparagus. Add the salt and pepper. If desired, sprinkle with the nutritional yeast.

TIP: *For a change of pace, you can substitute Homemade Garlic Mayonnaise (page 270) for the Dijon sauce.*

Per serving: 59 calories, 3 g protein, 8 g carbohydrates, 3 g total fat, 2 g saturated fat, 3 g fiber, 596 mg sodium

Homemade Garlic Mayonnaise

Prep Time: 5 minutes • Total Time: 20 minutes   Makes 12 servings

4–5 cloves garlic, crushed

1 egg yolk

1 tablespoon fresh lemon juice

¾ cup extra-virgin olive oil

¼ teaspoon salt (to taste)

¼ teaspoon ground black pepper (to taste)

1. Using a porcelain or marble mortar and pestle or a small food processor, pound or process the garlic to a paste. (Some small bits will not completely break down.) Alternately, mince the garlic very fine, then mash it well with the flat side of a cleaver or a large knife.

2. In a medium bowl, whisk the garlic with the egg yolk. Add the lemon juice and whisk to combine. Add the oil drop by drop at first, whisking constantly. After you have added about ¼ cup of the oil, drizzle in the rest in a thin stream, whisking constantly until the mayonnaise has emulsified.

3. Season with the salt and pepper, and add more lemon juice, if desired. Refrigerate the mayonnaise in a tightly covered glass jar for as long as a week. The flavor is best when the mayonnaise is fresh, but any left over is good in salads.

Per serving (1 tablespoon): 132 calories, 0 g protein, 0.5 g carbohydrates, 14 g total fat, 2 g saturated fat, 0 g fiber, 49 mg sodium

Roasted Asparagus

Prep Time: 5 minutes • Total Time: 20 minutes   Makes 4 servings

- 2 tablespoons coconut oil
- 2 bunches asparagus (about 30 spears), trimmed
- ¼ teaspoon salt
- ¼ teaspoon ground black pepper
- 2 tablespoons fresh lime juice (optional)

1. Preheat the oven to 350°F. Put the oil on a rimmed baking sheet. Place in the preheating oven for 1 minute, or until the oil melts. Remove the pan from the oven.

2. Toss the asparagus with the oil on the baking sheet. Sprinkle with the salt and pepper. Roast for 10 to 12 minutes, or until the asparagus is just tender-crisp. Don't overcook. Just before serving, add the lime juice and additional salt and pepper, if desired.

Per serving: 87 calories, 3 g protein, 6 g carbohydrates, 7 g total fat, 6 g saturated fat, 3 g fiber, 148 mg sodium

Crispy Roasted Kale Chips

Prep Time: 10 minutes • Total Time: 40 minutes   Makes 4 servings

2   bunches kale (about 2–2½ pounds), hard stems removed, finely chopped (about 9 cups chopped)

¼   cup coconut oil or extra-virgin olive oil

¼   teaspoon kosher salt

¼   teaspoon ground black pepper

½   teaspoon nutritional yeast (optional)

1. Preheat the oven to 375°F. Arrange 3 oven racks in each third of the oven.

2. In a large bowl, toss the kale with the oil, salt, and pepper. Arrange loosely on 3 baking sheets (or roast in batches). Roast for 15 minutes, or until crisp. Sprinkle with nutritional yeast, if desired.

TIP: *When arranging the kale on the baking sheets, be sure to allow a lot of space on each pan. If kale is arranged too closely, it will steam rather than roast and won't get crispy.*

Per serving: 194 calories, 6 protein, 13 g carbohydrates, 15 g total fat, 12 g saturated fat, 3 g fiber, 177 mg sodium

Homemade Hummus

Prep Time: 5 minutes • Total Time: 10 minutes   Makes 8 servings

1   can (15.5 ounces) chickpeas, rinsed and drained

3   cloves garlic, minced

3   tablespoons fresh lemon juice

½   cup water (or more to taste)

3   tablespoons tahini (sesame paste)

½–1 teaspoon ground cumin

2   teaspoons extra-virgin olive oil

Pinch of ground paprika (optional)

Pinch of ground red pepper (optional)

1. In the bowl of a food processor, combine the chickpeas, garlic, lemon juice, and water. Process for 1 minute, or until smooth. If too thick, add more water.

2. Add the tahini and cumin and stir to combine. Taste and add more lemon juice, tahini, or cumin if desired.

3. Spread the hummus into a shallow bowl and drizzle with the oil. Add paprika and ground red pepper, if desired.

TIP: *Hummus is delicious as a dip for vegetables or added to any salad for extra protein and healthy fat. Chickpeas, a whole food, are highly nutritious, supplying protein and fabulous complex carbohydrates.*

Per serving: 81 calories, 3 g protein, 8 g carbohydrates, 5 g total fat, 0.5 g saturated fat, 2 g fiber, 111 mg sodium

Chicken with Chickpeas and Artichokes

Prep Time: 20 minutes • Total Time: 1 hour 10 minutes   Makes 4 servings

1½ pounds boneless, skinless free-range chicken breasts, cut into 8 pieces

¼ teaspoon + ⅛ teaspoon sea salt

¼ teaspoon ground black pepper

3 tablespoons coconut oil

1 yellow onion, chopped

4–5 cloves garlic, thinly sliced

1 teaspoon ground turmeric

½ teaspoon ground cumin

½ teaspoon ground coriander

¼ teaspoon red-pepper flakes

1 cinnamon stick or ¼ teaspoon ground cinnamon

1 bay leaf

2 cups low-sodium organic chicken broth, divided

2 teaspoons grated lemon peel

3 tablespoons fresh lemon juice, divided

1 can (15 ounces) chickpeas, rinsed, drained, and tossed with 1 tablespoon lemon juice

1 can (14 ounces) artichoke hearts, rinsed and drained

2 tablespoons chopped fresh cilantro

1. Season the chicken with ¼ teaspoon of the salt and the pepper. In a Dutch oven or heavy pot over medium heat, heat the oil. Cook the chicken, working in batches if necessary, for 6 minutes, turning once, or until well browned on each side. Transfer to a plate and set aside.

2. Add the onion to the pot and cook for 5 minutes, or until soft and golden. Add the garlic and cook for 1 minute, stirring. Add the turmeric, cumin, coriander, pepper flakes, cinnamon, and bay leaf. Cook for 1 minute, stirring constantly.

3. Pour in ¼ cup of the broth to deglaze the pot, stirring to loosen any brown bits stuck to the bottom. Stir in the remaining ⅛ teaspoon salt and cook for 2 minutes, or until the liquid is absorbed. Stir in the remaining 1¾ cups broth, the lemon peel, and 2 tablespoons of the lemon juice. Reduce the heat to medium-low, cover, and simmer for 15 minutes.

4. Add the reserved chicken, the chickpeas, and artichoke hearts. Stir gently to combine. Increase the heat to medium-high and simmer, uncovered, for 10 min-

utes, stirring occasionally, or until the chicken is no longer pink. Stir in the remaining 1 tablespoon lemon juice. Remove and discard the cinnamon stick and bay leaf. Garnish with the cilantro.

TIP: *You can easily use firm white fish, such as halibut or grouper, cut into pieces, in place of the chicken. Begin the recipe by cooking the onion. Proceed as directed, but substitute vegetable broth for the chicken broth. Add the fish during the last 5 minutes of cooking.*

Per serving: 409 calories, 43 g protein, 22 g carbohydrates, 16 g total fat, 10 g saturated fat, 5 g fiber, 973 mg sodium

Spicy Chicken with Sautéed Greens

Prep Time: 5 minutes • Total Time: 30 minutes   Makes 4 servings

4 boneless, skinless free-range chicken breasts (6 ounces each)	1 large sweet onion, thinly sliced
1½ teaspoons ground cumin	1 large bunch collard greens, kale, or chard, thick stems removed (about 1 pound trimmed)
¼ teaspoon ground red pepper	
½ teaspoon salt, divided	⅛ teaspoon ground black pepper
2 tablespoons coconut oil, divided	

1. Heat the oven to 400°F. Season the chicken with the cumin, red pepper, and ¼ teaspoon of the salt.

2. In a large skillet over medium heat, heat 1 tablespoon of the oil. Cook the chicken for 8 minutes, turning once, or until browned on both sides. Transfer the chicken to a roasting pan and bake for 6 minutes, or until a thermometer inserted in the thickest portion of a breast registers 165°F and the juices run clear.

3. Return the skillet to medium heat and add the remaining 1 tablespoon oil. Cook the onion for 6 minutes, stirring frequently, or until translucent.

4. Meanwhile, thinly slice the greens crosswise. Add to the skillet and cook for 3 minutes, or until just tender. Season with the black pepper and remaining ¼ teaspoon salt. Transfer to a serving platter and top with the chicken.

Per serving: 316 calories, 39 g protein, 13 g carbohydrates, 12 g total fat, 7 g saturated fat, 3 g fiber, 523 mg sodium

Simple Thai Chicken Curry

Prep Time: 5 minutes • Total Time: 15 minutes   Makes 4 servings

- 1 teaspoon curry powder
- 1 teaspoon finely chopped red chile pepper or ½ teaspoon red-pepper flakes
- 1 tablespoon finely chopped lemongrass
- 1 pound boneless, skinless free-range chicken breasts, sliced
- 3 tablespoons coconut oil
- ½ cup canned coconut milk
- ½ cup salted peanut halves or cashew halves
- ⅛ teaspoon salt
- ⅛ teaspoon ground black pepper
- ½ cup roughly chopped cilantro

1. On a plate, combine the curry powder, chile pepper or pepper flakes, and lemongrass. Mix well. Coat the chicken slices with the curry mixture.

2. In a large skillet over medium heat, heat the oil. Cook the chicken for 4 minutes, turning occasionally, or until no longer pink and the juices run clear. Add the coconut milk and cook for 2 to 3 minutes, or until heated through. Add the nuts, salt, and pepper and cook for 30 seconds. Garnish with the cilantro before serving.

Per serving: 355 calories, 28 g protein, 5 g carbohydrates, 26 g total fat, 15 g saturated fat, 1 g fiber, 270 mg sodium

Chicken and Wild Mushrooms with Truffle Oil

Prep Time: 10 minutes • Total Time: 30 minutes   Makes 6 servings

3   tablespoons coconut oil, ghee, or organic butter, divided

2   pounds chicken tenders

1   pound assorted sliced mushrooms, such as shiitake, porcini, and cremini

6   whole cloves garlic

5   sprigs fresh thyme

¼   cup Marsala wine or dry sherry

2   cups organic chicken broth

1   cup white wine

¼   teaspoon kosher salt

¼   teaspoon ground black pepper

2   tablespoons truffle oil

1   tablespoon unsalted organic butter

1   recipe Quinoa with Lemon and Pine Nuts (page 249), optional

1. In a medium skillet over medium heat, heat 2 tablespoons of the oil, ghee, or butter. Cook the chicken in batches for 3 minutes, turning once, or until golden and just barely pink. Transfer to a plate and set aside.

2. In the same skillet over medium heat, heat the remaining 1 tablespoon oil, ghee, or butter. Cook the mushrooms, garlic, and thyme for 5 minutes, stirring occasionally, or until the mushrooms are golden brown. Stir in the Marsala or sherry, scraping up any brown bits on the bottom of the pan. Add the broth, white wine, salt, and pepper and bring to a boil. Add the reserved chicken. Simmer for 3 to 4 minutes, or until the liquid is reduced by half and the chicken is no longer pink. Stir in the truffle oil and unsalted butter. Serve over Quinoa with Lemon and Pine Nuts, if desired.

Per serving: 366 calories, 35 g protein, 8 g carbohydrates, 18 g total fat, 8 g saturated fat, 1 g fiber, 455 mg sodium

Easy Chicken with White Beans and Arugula

Prep Time: 15 minutes • Total Time: 1 hour   Makes 4 servings

MARINADE AND CHICKEN

- 2 tablespoons red wine vinegar
- 2 tablespoons chopped fresh thyme or rosemary
- 4 cloves garlic, minced
- 3 tablespoons extra-virgin olive oil
- $\frac{1}{4}$ teaspoon kosher salt
- $\frac{1}{4}$ teaspoon ground black pepper
- 4 boneless, skinless free-range chicken breasts (6 ounces each)
- 2 tablespoons coconut oil or organic butter

DRESSING

- 2 tablespoons extra-virgin olive oil
- 2 teaspoons Dijon mustard
- $\frac{1}{4}$ teaspoon salt
- $\frac{1}{4}$ teaspoon ground black pepper
- 6 cups arugula
- 1 can (15 ounces) white beans, rinsed and drained
- $\frac{1}{4}$ small red onion, thinly sliced (optional)

1. *To make the marinade:* In a large bowl, whisk together the vinegar, thyme or rosemary, garlic, oil, salt, and pepper. Add the chicken and toss to coat. Cover and refrigerate for 30 minutes or overnight.

2. *To make the dressing:* In a large bowl, whisk together the oil, mustard, salt, and pepper. Add the arugula, beans, and onion (if desired). Toss to coat.

3. In a large skillet over medium heat, heat the oil or butter. Remove the chicken from the marinade and cook for 12 to 16 minutes, turning once, or until a thermometer inserted in the thickest portion of a breast registers 165°F and the juices run clear. Serve the chicken with the arugula and bean salad.

Per serving: 508 calories, 42 g protein, 18 g carbohydrates, 29 g total fat, 10 g saturated fat, 4 g fiber, 509 mg sodium

One-Pot Chicken with Garlic and Winter Vegetables

Prep Time: 30 minutes • Total Time: 2 hours 10 minutes **Makes 8 servings**

3 tablespoons coconut oil, ghee, or organic butter, divided

2 sweet potatoes, peeled and cubed

12 shallots

8 carrots, quartered

4 parsnips, peeled and quartered

1 butternut squash, peeled and cubed (2 pounds)

1 turnip, peeled and quartered

4 ribs celery, sliced

4 large heads garlic, cloves separated

¼ teaspoon salt, divided

¼ teaspoon ground black pepper, divided

3 sprigs fresh thyme

1 cup chopped parsley

2 sprigs fresh rosemary

1 tablespoon lemon peel

1 organic, free-range chicken, cut up (about 4 pounds)

1 cup organic chicken broth

½ cup white wine

1. Preheat the oven to 350°F. In a large skillet over medium heat, heat 2 tablespoons of the oil, ghee, or butter. Cook the sweet potatoes, shallots, carrots, parsnips, squash, turnip, celery, garlic, ⅛ teaspoon of the salt, and ⅛ teaspoon of the pepper until the vegetables are golden brown on all sides. If necessary, do this in batches. Spoon into a large Dutch oven or any large, heavy lidded pot, and add the thyme, parsley, rosemary, and lemon peel. Stir to combine.

2. Return the skillet to medium heat, and heat the remaining 1 tablespoon oil, ghee, or butter. Cook the chicken until brown on all sides. Season with the remaining ¼ teaspoon salt and ¼ teaspoon pepper. Transfer to the Dutch oven and surround with the vegetables.

3. In a small bowl, combine the broth and wine and pour over the chicken and vegetables. Cover and bake for 55 minutes, or until a thermometer inserted in the thickest portion of the chicken registers 165°F and the meat is no longer pink.

Per serving: 732 calories, 44 g protein, 65 g carbohydrates, 34 g total fat, 13 g saturated fat, 8 g fiber, 378 mg sodium

Salmon in Parchment

Prep Time: 20 minutes • Total Time: 35 minutes　　　　　　　　　　Makes 4 servings

- 2 ribs organic celery, cut into matchsticks
- 2 organic carrots, cut into matchsticks
- 2 organic leeks, cut into matchsticks
- 4 wild-caught salmon steaks (6 ounces each)
- 1 tablespoon coconut oil
- 2 cups organic spinach leaves
- 1/4 cup dry white wine
- 2 tablespoons fresh lemon juice
- 1 bottle (8 ounces) clam juice
- 1 large tomato, chopped
- 1 tablespoon chopped fresh tarragon or thyme
- 1/4 teaspoon ground black pepper

1. Preheat the oven to 375°F. Bring a large pot of water to a boil. Blanch the celery, carrots, and leeks for 1 minute. Rinse under cold water and drain. Set aside.

2. Cut 4 pieces of parchment paper, each 30" long. Cut each piece into a heart shape for easy folding. Brush each steak with the oil. Lay 1/2 cup of the spinach leaves on one side of a piece of parchment. Top with one-quarter of the blanched vegetables. Place a salmon steak on the top. Repeat with the remaining spinach, vegetables, and salmon.

3. In a small bowl, combine the wine, lemon juice, and clam juice. Drizzle the mixture over the salmon packets. Divide the tomato and tarragon or thyme among the packets. Sprinkle with the pepper. Fold over and crimp the edges to close the packets. Place on a baking sheet and bake for 15 minutes, or until the salmon is opaque.

Per serving: 314 calories, 32 g protein, 14 g carbohydrates, 13 g total fat, 4 g saturated fat, 3 g fiber, 255 mg sodium

Simple Roasted Wild Salmon Fillets

Prep Time: 5 minutes • Total Time: 50 minutes   Makes 4 servings

4   wild-caught salmon fillets
    (6 ounces each)

1   tablespoon fresh lemon juice

2   teaspoons coconut oil, butter,
    or ghee

¼   teaspoon salt

¼   teaspoon ground black pepper

1. In a glass baking dish, arrange the salmon fillets. Sprinkle with the lemon juice and let stand for 30 minutes at room temperature.

2. Preheat the oven to 425°F. Brush the oil, butter, or ghee on the fish and season with the salt and pepper. Bake for 15 to 20 minutes, or until the fish is opaque.

Per serving: 296 calories, 39 g protein, 0.5 g carbohydrates, 15 g total fat, 4 g saturated fat, 0 g fiber, 230 mg sodium

Grilled Thai-Style Fish

Prep Time: 10 minutes • Total Time: 40 minutes   Makes 4 servings

1   cup canned unsweetened coconut
    milk (not light)

2   tablespoons fresh lime juice

1   tablespoon minced fresh ginger

2   cloves garlic, minced

    Pinch of ground red pepper

¼   cup chopped fresh cilantro, divided

¼   cup finely chopped scallions, divided

¼   teaspoon salt (to taste)

¼   teaspoon ground black pepper
    (to taste)

4   mahi mahi, monchong, or onaga
    fillets (6 ounces each)

1   tablespoon coconut oil, organic
    ghee, or butter

1. Preheat the grill to medium-high heat. In a medium skillet, combine the coconut milk, lime juice, ginger, garlic, and red pepper. Bring to a boil. Reduce the heat to a simmer and cook for 10 minutes, stirring constantly, or until the sauce thickens slightly and is reduced to about ¾ cup. Remove from the heat. Add half of the cilantro and half of the scallions and stir to combine. Season with the salt and black pepper.

2. Brush the fish on both sides with the oil, ghee, or butter and ¼ cup of the coconut sauce. Grill for 10 to 14 minutes, turning once, or until it flakes easily and grill marks appear. Serve with the remaining sauce drizzled on top. Sprinkle with the remaining cilantro and scallions.

TIP: *Monchong is also known as Hawaiian black bass, and onaga is also known as Hawaiian red snapper.*

Per serving: 293 calories, 33 g protein, 4 g carbohydrates, 17 g total fat, 14 g saturated fat, 1 g fiber, 304 mg sodium

Mahi Mahi in Cilantro Curry Sauce

Prep Time: 10 minutes • Total Time: 25 minutes   Makes 4 servings

- 2 tablespoons coconut oil
- 1½ pounds mahi mahi or other white fish
- ½ cup canned coconut milk
- 1 small bunch cilantro
- 2 large cloves garlic, sliced
- 3 spring onions, chopped
- 1½ tablespoons curry powder
- 1 cup vegetable or fish stock
- 2 tablespoons fresh lime juice

1. In a large skillet over medium heat, heat the oil. Sear the fish for 2 to 4 minutes, turning once, or until golden on both sides. Transfer to a plate and set aside.

2. In a blender or food processor, combine the coconut milk, cilantro, garlic, onions, curry powder, and stock. Blend or process until smooth. Return the skillet to medium-high heat. Transfer the coconut milk mixture to the skillet and cook for 2 minutes. Add the lime juice and reserved fish. Simmer for 5 minutes, or until the fish flakes easily. Serve the fish with the sauce spooned over the top.

Per serving: 281 calories, 33 g protein, 5 g carbohydrates, 14 g total fat, 12 g saturated fat, 2 g fiber, 296 mg sodium

Gingered Red Snapper

Prep Time: 10 minutes • Total Time: 45 minutes   Makes 4 servings

- 4 ounces fresh ginger, thinly sliced and cut into fine matchsticks
- ¼ cup fresh lime juice
- 2½ tablespoons coconut oil
- 6 cloves garlic, thinly sliced
- 1 cup canned coconut milk
- 1½ teaspoons sesame seeds
- 2 tablespoons soy sauce
- 4 red snapper fillets (6 ounces each)
- Fresh cilantro, for garnish
- Fresh Italian parsley, for garnish

1. Preheat the oven to 350°F or a grill to medium-high heat. In a medium bowl, combine the ginger and lime juice. Let the mixture stand for 10 minutes at room temperature.

2. In a heavy skillet over medium heat, heat the oil. Cook the garlic for 3 minutes, or until soft and golden. Add the coconut milk and cook, stirring, until heated through. Transfer to the bowl with the ginger mixture and stir to combine.

3. In a dry skillet over medium heat, toast the sesame seeds for 2 to 3 minutes, stirring frequently, or until golden. Stir in the soy sauce. Transfer to the bowl and stir to combine the sauce.

4. On each of 4 pieces of foil, arrange 1 fillet and top with the sauce. Fold over and crimp the edges to form packets. Arrange the packets on the grill or arrange on a baking sheet and put in the oven. Grill or bake for 12 to 15 minutes, or until the fish flakes easily but is still moist. Remove from the foil and garnish with the cilantro and parsley.

Per serving: 417 calories, 37 g protein, 10 g carbohydrates, 23 g total fat, 19 g saturated fat, 2 g fiber, 537 mg sodium

Cinnamon Baked Apples with Pecans

Prep Time: 5 minutes • Total Time: 20 minutes   Makes 4 servings

4 Granny Smith apples, sliced in halves or quarters

2 cups unsweetened cranberry juice

2 teaspoons coconut oil, at room temperature

2 teaspoons ground cinnamon

⅔ cup pecan halves

1. Preheat the oven to 350°F. Place the apples in a baking dish and pour the juice over them. Dot with the oil and sprinkle with the cinnamon.

2. Bake for 15 minutes, basting with the juice (as it heats, it will become syrupy), or until soft but not mushy. Serve topped with the pecans and syrup from the pan.

Per serving: 252 calories, 2 g protein, 38 g carbohydrates, 13 g total fat, 3 g saturated fat, 5 g fiber, 4 mg sodium

The Ultimate Green Smoothie

Prep Time: 10 minutes • Total Time: 15 minutes   Makes 2 servings

1 cup water	¼ cup frozen organic blueberries
3½ cups chopped organic spinach, Swiss chard, or kale	¼ cup frozen organic raspberries
½ cup parsley	1 tablespoon ground flax seeds
1 banana	2 tablespoons hemp or grass-fed, organic whey protein (optional)
1 pear or 1 apple, cored and chopped	

In a blender, combine the water and spinach, Swiss chard, or kale. Blend on high speed for 30 seconds to 1 minute, or until smooth. Add the parsley, banana, pear or apple, blueberries, raspberries, flax seeds, and whey protein. Blend on high speed for 1 minute, or until thoroughly blended.

TIP: For an extra-thick and creamy smoothie, use a frozen banana.

Per serving: 202 calories, 13 g protein, 36 g carbohydrates, 3 g total fat, 0.5 g saturated fat, 8 g fiber, 57 mg sodium

Power Smoothie

Prep Time: 10 minutes • Total Time: 15 minutes   Makes 2 servings

1 cup water	1 organic apple, cored and chopped
2 cups chopped organic kale	½ cup frozen organic berries
1 cup chopped cilantro	1 tablespoon ground flax seeds
1 orange, peeled, sectioned, and chopped	2 tablespoons hemp or grass-fed, organic whey protein (optional)

In a blender, combine the water and kale. Blend on high speed for 1 minute, or until smooth. Add the cilantro, orange, apple, berries, flax seeds, and whey protein. Blend on high speed for 1 minute, or until thoroughly blended.

Per serving: 196 calories, 14 g protein, 34 g carbohydrates, 3 g total fat, 0 g saturated fat, 7 g fiber, 37 mg sodium

Super Smoothie

Prep Time: 10 minutes • Total Time: 15 minutes

Makes 2 servings

½	cup water	1	organic apple, cored and chopped
2	cups chopped Swiss chard	¾	cup organic strawberries
2	cups parsley	2	tablespoons ground flax seeds
1	banana, frozen	2	tablespoons hemp or grass-fed, organic whey protein (optional)

In a blender, combine the water, Swiss chard, parsley, banana, apple, strawberries, flax seeds, and whey protein. Blend on high speed for 1 to 2 minutes, or until thoroughly blended.

Per serving: 232 calories, 14 g protein, 40 g carbohydrates, 4 g total fat, 0.5 g saturated fat, 9 g fiber, 117 mg sodium

Purple Power Smoothie

Prep Time: 10 minutes • Total Time: 15 minutes   Makes 2 servings

½ cup water

2 cups chopped purple kale

1 mango, peeled and diced

¼ cup frozen organic blueberries

¼ cup frozen organic raspberries

½ cup acai juice

2 tablespoons ground flax seeds

2 tablespoons hemp or grass-fed, organic whey protein (optional)

In a blender, combine the water, kale, mango, blueberries, raspberries, acai juice, flax seeds, and whey protein. Blend on high speed for 1 to 2 minutes, or until thoroughly blended.

Per serving: 268 calories, 15 g protein, 47 g carbohydrates, 5 g total fat, 0.5 g saturated fat, 7 g fiber, 36 mg sodium

Asian Smoothie

Prep Time: 10 minutes • Total Time: 15 minutes   Makes 2 servings

1 cup chilled water	1 tablespoon lime juice
3½ cups organic spinach	1 teaspoon chopped fresh ginger
3–4 leaves bok choy or Chinese cabbage	2 tablespoons ground flax seeds
1 apple, cored and chopped	2 tablespoons hemp or grass-fed, organic whey protein (optional)

In a blender, combine the water and spinach. Blend on high speed for 30 seconds to 1 minute, or until smooth. Add the bok choy or Chinese cabbage, apple, lime juice, ginger, flax seeds, and whey protein. Blend on high speed for 1 to 2 minutes, or until thoroughly blended.

Per serving: 149 calories, 12 g protein, 19 g carbohydrates, 4 g total fat, 0.5 g saturated fat, 6 g fiber, 63 mg sodium

Ginger Smoothie

Prep Time: 10 minutes • Total Time: 15 minutes   Makes 2 servings

1½ cups water

3½ cups spinach

2 cups chopped kale

2 leaves bok choy

2 teaspoons chopped fresh ginger

1 banana, frozen

1 carrot, chopped

1 pear, cored and chopped

2 tablespoons ground flax seeds

¼ cup organic raspberries

¼ cup organic blueberries

2 tablespoons hemp or grass-fed, organic whey protein (optional)

In a blender, combine the water, spinach, and kale. Blend on high speed for 1 minute, or until smooth. Add the bok choy, ginger, banana, carrot, pear, flax seeds, raspberries, blueberries, and whey protein. Blend on high speed for 1 to 2 minutes, or until thoroughly blended.

Per serving: 260 calories, 16 g protein, 46 g carbohydrates, 5 g total fat, 0 g saturated fat, 11 g fiber, 110 mg sodium

Sassy Smoothie

Prep Time: 10 minutes • Total Time: 15 minutes   Makes 2 servings

1 cup chilled water

2 cups chopped kale

3½ cups chopped spinach or Swiss chard

1 cup chopped cilantro

2 teaspoons chopped fresh ginger

1 banana

1 pear, cored and chopped

1 seedless orange, peeled and chopped

1 tablespoon ground flax seeds

2 tablespoons hemp or grass-fed, organic whey protein (optional)

In a blender, combine the water, kale, spinach or Swiss chard, cilantro, ginger, banana, pear, orange, flax seeds, and whey protein. Blend on high speed for 1 to 2 minutes, or until thoroughly blended.

Per serving: 250 calories, 16 g protein, 46 g carbohydrates, 3 g total fat, 0 g saturated fat, 10 g fiber, 79 mg sodium

The LiverUp! Diaries

TRACY ULMER, 49

It's Changed My Life

Lost: 13 pounds

Blood sugar, iron count, cholesterol: Normal

Carb cravings: Gone

Hot flashes: Disappeared

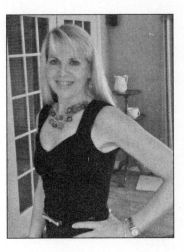

Just a few years ago, I was making my way through menopause, teaching yoga, and living the busy life of a mother of three. My hot flashes were worse than ever, coming on 15 to 20 times a day. I could never predict when one would come next, and that made me so anxious that I had my heart checked. At the time, I drank homemade iced tea throughout my day and experienced intense carb cravings. I would find my blood sugars fluctuating throughout my day from high to low. (I was in tune with sugar reactions because I'd had gestational diabetes during my pregnancies.)

These were just little glitches in my life, though. I always thought of myself as a very healthy person and was comfortable with my weight. I decided to do the LiverUp! Cleanse when a friend told me about it. I wanted to do something good for myself—the idea of cleansing toxins from my body sounded great to me.

I never expected the cleanse to change my life, but that's what it did. Cutting out caffeinated iced tea was really hard—for 4 days, it felt like I was slogging through mud with a foggy brain! But after that I noticed my cravings and hot flashes had almost disappeared. By the end of the cleanse I'd dropped 13 pounds, and I've dropped even more since. I have so much more energy and an overall sense of well-being that I didn't have before. I'm told I look younger, and I definitely feel younger. The blood work from my recent physical came back with all normal levels for iron count, sugar, and cholesterol.

I used to feel that being tired was part of getting older. Now I'm energized, tuned into my body, and inspired to eat mindfully. I eat the way the cleanse taught me, with a new appreciation for a variety of foods. The cleanse changed my life completely.

CHAPTER 10

Easing Back, Moving Forward

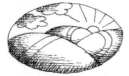

Now that you've arrived at the end of your LiverUp! Cleanse, take a moment to reflect on your experience. Over these past 12 days, you've turned your thoughts and your intentions toward your physical, emotional, and spiritual well-being. You've detoxed your liver and cleaned your gut with healing foods and, perhaps, a fast. You've helped your body release the many toxins it's been storing.

At the same time, you've been gathering information about yourself. Especially if you've been journaling, you've been collecting your own empirical evidence about the way you feel when you eat whole, clean foods. You've begun to learn which foods feed you physically, emotionally, and spiritually—and which ones don't.

Cleansing offers you the gift of waking up and the chance to pay attention to all that is happening in the present moment. It's given you the opportunity to be intentional—about what, when, and how you eat; about how you move through your day; about when you turn out the lights to enjoy restful, restorative sleep. Cleansing gives you a moment in time to pause, reflect, and intentionally choose the way you want to live your life, rather than impulsively reacting to each curveball life throws at you.

While so much of life is far beyond your control, the way you respond is within your own power. And the way you respond, based on the choices you make, affects the way you feel physically, emotionally, and spiritually.

Think of the many choices you've made during your LiverUp! Cleanse:

You've been eating fresh, vital, and healing foods; hydrating your body; allowing yourself to rest; practicing deep breathing; and committing to exercise. All of these choices promise to bring you to a new level of health in mind, body, and spirit. Over the past 12 days, you've given yourself a gift of self-care, something that often seems in short supply when life demands much of us. There's always a reasonable excuse *not* to take care of ourselves. Mostly, we convince ourselves that everyone else's needs must come first—and that leaves us with little to no energy or compassion to offer ourselves. And when this happens, we tend to reach for comfort foods that sabotage our health and well-being.

The 12 days of your cleanse, while rewarding—and, I hope, joyful—are intense, and when they're over, you may be eager to get back to "normal." As you gently ease back into your daily rhythm, how will you honor your commitment to this journey toward whole-body health and healing? The good news is that there's a way to take the lessons you've learned and the new habits you've acquired and find ways to fit them into your everyday life. That's what this final chapter is all about.

Begin at the Beginning

When you begin with food, noticing how it affects your body, mind, and spirit, you become much more present to your life because you are more energized, clear-thinking, and balanced emotionally. As you experience more vitality, you become willing to return to those behaviors that attune you to nature's daily and seasonal rhythms. The result? You're more aligned with your true inner nature and are more connected with all that surrounds you. You feel more whole.

That's why the LiverUp! Cleanse begins with food. But it doesn't end there. Committing to a whole-life approach to health—as you nourish your body, mind, and spirit—can help bring about whole-body healing.

Each of us has a different rhythm and pace to our days, to our lives. And each of us has our own individual challenges. But no matter where you are or what challenges are before you, the most important thing is to honor yourself and your intention to participate joyfully in the present moment. You can acknowledge that change is the only constant—and that allows you to relax and let life flow through you, just as your breath does. You don't have to struggle so hard. You don't have to push against the current.

Observe your thoughts. Notice how you're feeling. Try to release your self-judgment and stay in the moment. Come back to your breath. The thoughts and feelings will pass. They always do.

Cleansing teaches you to pause and breathe, to inhale life-giving oxygen, and release anything that's not serving you in the moment. Simply and profoundly, your breath serves, in every moment, as a reminder that you need to remain open to—and to accept—life as it is.

Each breath is a spiritual practice. Allowing yourself to experience the moment—letting it all in physically, mentally, and emotionally and in turn releasing that which you've held within, clearly expressing your feelings, thoughts, and perceptions—is a spiritual practice that bathes your heart and mind. In short, it sets you free to live life on life's terms.

The key is to stay awake. Stay with the eating strategies that have worked best for you as you ease into normal eating. Listen to your body's voice. The more you stay on your path toward health and wholeness, the clearer that voice will become.

Moving On

As you move forward, see what you can take with you from this cleansing experience. It may not have anything to do with food. It may be something you learned about yourself along the way. It may be that you're willing to honor your body—and your life—in a new way. It may be that you want to take just a few minutes every day to sit quietly. See page 298 for easy ways to weave the cleanse into your life.

Clean food helps to create a clean body. A clean body helps create a clean, healthy way of living. Clean thoughts help create gratitude and loving kindness. Loving kindness helps to change the world. Share your gratitude and you will find peace.

Choose Your Healthy Life

Think of the chart that follows as a guide—not as a prescription. Each day, try to choose one or two suggestions from each section—more, if you like—and see how they fit into your new postcleanse life. Mix and match, and see what works best for you.

Nourish Your Body with Healthy, Whole Foods
Eat nutrient-dense whole foods—those that look the same on your plate as they do when they're growing—just as nature made them. These are naturally rich in vitamins, minerals, fiber, and healthy fats.
Fill your plate with vegetables. The more dark green ones, the better—think kale, collards, broccoli, cabbage, and Brussels sprouts.
As often as you can, buy organic vegetables and fruits—this is especially important for fruits and veggies on the "Dirty Dozen" list. (See list on page 94.)
Eat fewer conventionally raised animal products. According to the EPA, meat and dairy products contain higher levels of pesticides than plant foods.[1] In addition, most conventionally raised animals require some antibiotics, drugs, or hormones. Many of these chemicals are fat-soluble, accumulating in the animals' milk, meat, and fatty tissue. Growth hormones and antibiotics are also serious concerns and are invariably found in commercial milk, cheese, and butter. It's not always be easy to find organic products, but the tips found at eatwild.com will help you get started.
Eat a variety of protein foods daily, including blue-green algae, spirulina, free-range eggs, organic whey powder, wild-caught smaller fish (mahi mahi, halibut, striped bass, salmon), and, if you choose to eat meat, select among pastured, grass-fed animals.
Eat healthy fats—coconut oil, flax seeds, chia seeds, extra-virgin organic olive oil, and butter made from the milk of grass-fed cows. These fats help balance blood sugar and brain function, reduce inflammation, lower triglycerides, and keep you feeling full (see Chapter 5).
Drink half your body weight in ounces of water each day, starting your day with lemon and water. Remember that lemon water supports your liver, colon, and kidneys, helping to flush toxins out of your body all day long.

Avoid processed, refined foods with an ingredient list that includes white flour, sugar (especially high-fructose corn syrup), preservatives, or unhealthy fats. These can trigger the release of insulin, burden your liver's two-phase detoxification process, and increase your body's toxic load.

Minimize alcohol and coffee consumption. Your liver is the only organ that metabolizes alcohol, converting it into sugar for energy or storing it as fat when there's too much. When it's stored as fat, alcohol can act like an irritant to your liver. Both alcohol and coffee can trigger the release of cortisol, the stress hormone secreted by the adrenal glands that signals danger.

Nourish Your Mind and Spirit

Commit to getting more sleep. Turn off all electronic screens an hour before lights-out (unless it's a device made specifically for reading). Dim the lights and read for 30 minutes or so before you turn in.

Practice deep breathing and meditation. Meditation allows you a growing understanding of your mind, your choices, your thoughts, words, and actions—and their connection to your sense of peace and well-being. Choose a time and place to show up for your practice, and commit to a specific duration—perhaps 5, 10, or 20 minutes. Make sure it's an amount of time you can realistically manage.

Journal about your meditation practice. Ask yourself, in writing, about any roadblocks that may be preventing you from a consistent practice. Whatever they are—a lack of time; a host of obligations, priorities, and responsibilities; or an unwillingness to care for yourself—they are universal, and often constant.

Get outside. Breathe. Walk around the block or take a walk in nature, if you can. Fresh air and movement bring oxygen to your cells, rejuvenating your whole body.

Roll out your yoga mat. Yoga massages your internal organs, helping your body to flush out excess fluids. Along with walking, it brings fresh blood that contains nutrients and oxygen.

MARTHA VICTOR, 54

A Process of Discovery

Lost: 8 pounds

Coffee habit: Conquered

Sleep: Better than ever

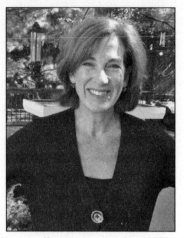

This cleanse came at the perfect time for me. Losing my job the week before could have put me in a depression mode, feeling like I didn't have control over much at all. If it weren't for the cleanse, I'm quite sure I would have proceeded with my coffee, a couple of glasses of wine every night, snacking, and not sleeping well.

The cleanse has changed my life in many ways. I didn't miss coffee, sugar, gluten, or wine one bit—in fact, I never noticed any of them were gone. In addition, I have always attributed stress to the 2 extra pounds I have that seem to come and go. But though I didn't need—or expect—to lose a single pound, I lost 8 pounds. I learned so much about healthy foods and enjoyed my daily trek to the market. I discovered things I never knew existed! Before the cleanse, I had never heard of nut butters or coconut oil.

I feel so much healthier and no longer need an occasional sleep aid to help me get 6 hours of sleep. I sleep a full 8 hours a night! Now I'll have wine on weekends only, and I won't go back to caffeine. Though I'll drink decaf because I love the taste, coffee is no longer a habit. And because I suddenly had so much energy, I really got into the habit of exercising. I still work out every day.

I've been a lifetime Weight Watchers member since 1981 and am meticulous about tracking every single thing that I eat. With the cleanse, though, I never tracked a thing and loved the fact that I was consuming so many good-for-my-body foods that it didn't make a difference if I ate 2 ounces or a whole bowlful. For me, the cleanse was a lovely experience.

APPENDIX

Heal Your Whole Body *Sample Menu Plans*

Here are some suggested meal plans for your LiverUp! 12-day cleanse. Because your liver craves raw vegetables and fruit, many of the recipes you'll find in Chapter 9 are raw. Remember: Leafy vegetables—in a beautiful array of colors—and fresh fruits contain living enzymes, natural antioxidants, and chlorophyll that cleanse your bowel and heal your liver. Plus, raw vegetables and fruits reduce excess acidity in your body, and that helps reduce inflammation.

You can follow these menu plans exactly as they are, using the recipes in Chapter 9, to make the cleanse super-easy. Or you can get creative. Pull out your cookbooks, comb the Internet—then see what's available at your local market and have fun cooking. Just follow the guidelines on pages 91–92 to be sure you're getting all of the nutrients you need for the most beneficial, healing cleanse possible.

Be sure to start each day with your lemon water—and hydrate frequently throughout the day. Remember: Drink half your body weight in ounces every single day. (So if you weigh 150 pounds, drink 75 ounces of water daily.) And don't forget your daily cup of dandelion root tea as well as your milk thistle supplement.

Most of all, enjoy your LiverUp! Cleanse. I'd love to hear from you about your experience. You can find me at mindfullyfed.com. Be well!

Sample Menus

Wake Up
Drink 2 large glasses of purified water with the juice of half a lemon, lime, or orange.**

Breakfast
2 poached eggs over sautéed kale with flax seeds

1 cup berries

Dandelion root or kukicha tea

Morning Snack
Ultimate Green Smoothie *(page 286)*

Lunch
Salmon Avocado Wrap, made with broccoli sprouts *(page 245)*

Kimchi *(page 261)*

Afternoon Snack
¼ cup raw pumpkin seeds (pepitas)

Dinner
Simple Thai Chicken Curry *(page 275)*

Roasted Brussels Sprouts with Caramelized Onions *(page 264)*

After-Dinner Snack
½ cup berries

Herb tea

Wake Up
Drink 2 large glasses of purified water with the juice of half a lemon, lime, or orange.**

Breakfast
Ultimate Green Smoothie *(page 286)*

Dandelion root or kukicha tea

Morning Snack
8 walnut halves

Herbal tea

Lunch
Gazpacho *(page 254)* in warmer months or
Simply Divine Pureed Cauliflower Soup *(page 258)*
Watercress Salad *(page 231)*

Afternoon Snack
Organic vegetable or V8 juice (add nutritional yeast flakes* if desired)

Dinner
Salmon in Parchment *(page 280)*
Arugula and Pear Salad *(page 239)*
Roasted Asparagus *(page 271)*

After-Dinner Snack
½ cup berries
Herbal tea

DAY 3

Wake Up
Drink 2 large glasses of purified water with the juice of half a lemon, lime, or orange.**

Breakfast
2 sautéed (over-easy) eggs over sautéed organic spinach, chard, or kale with flax seeds
Dandelion root or kukicha tea

Morning Snack
½ cup raw pumpkin seeds
Herbal tea

Lunch
Ultimate Green Smoothie *(page 286)*
Quinoa Porridge *(page 228)*

Afternoon Snack
Crispy Roasted Kale Chips *(page 272)*

Dinner
Chicken with Chickpeas and Artichokes *(page 276)*
Cabbage and Daikon Salad with Sprouts *(page 236)*

After-Dinner Snack
½ cup berries

Herbal tea

DAY 4

Wake Up
Drink 2 large glasses of purified water with the juice of half a lemon, lime, or orange.**

Breakfast
2 sautéed (over-easy) eggs over sautéed spinach, chard, kale, collards, or dandelion greens with flax seeds

Dandelion root or kukicha tea

Morning Snack
Smoothie of choice *(pages 286 to 292)*

Lunch
Broccoli and Fennel Soup *(page 253)*

Lentil Salad *(page 230)*

Afternoon Snack
1 cup jicama slices

Dinner
Kale, Squash, and White Bean Salad *(page 243)*

Dandelion Greens with Hot Olive Oil Dressing *(page 229)*

After-Dinner Snack
½ cup berries

Herbal tea

DAY 5

Wake Up
Drink 2 large glasses of purified water with the juice of half a lemon, lime, or orange.**

Breakfast
Ultimate Green Smoothie *(page 286)*

Morning Snack
8 walnut halves

Dandelion root or kukicha tea

Lunch

Watercress Soup *(page 252)*

Curried Quinoa and Chickpea Lettuce Wraps *(page 246)*

Afternoon Snack

Cut-up vegetables (carrots; celery; cucumbers; radishes; snap peas; red, yellow, orange, or green peppers) with 2 ounces hummus

Dinner

Roasted Cauliflower, Broccolini, and Chickpeas *(page 263)*

Kale Slaw with Red Cabbage and Carrots *(page 266)*

After-Dinner Snack

Cinnamon Baked Apples with Pecans *(page 285)*

Herbal tea

DAY 6

Wake Up

Drink 2 large glasses of purified water with the juice of half a lemon, lime, or orange.**

Breakfast

2 poached eggs over sautéed kale with flax seeds

1 cup berries

Dandelion root or kukicha tea

Morning Snack

8 walnut halves

Lunch

Hearty Cleansing Soup *(page 251)*

Afternoon Snack

Organic vegetable or V8 juice (can add nutritional yeast flakes* if desired)

Dinner

Arugula, Pomegranate, and Pecan Salad *(page 237)*

After-Dinner Snack

$\frac{1}{2}$ cup berries

Herbal tea

Wake Up
Drink 2 large glasses of purified water with the juice of half a lemon, lime, or orange.**

Breakfast
Ultimate Green Smoothie *(page 286)*

Dandelion root or kukicha tea

Morning Snack
12 almonds

Lunch
Avocado Egg Salad Wraps *(page 247)*

Kimchi *(page 261)*

Afternoon Snack
Crispy Roasted Kale Chips *(page 272)*

Dinner
Moroccan Quinoa *(page 248)*

Autumn Arugula Salad *(page 234)*

After-Dinner Snack
¹⁄₂ cup berries

Herbal tea

DAY 8 (OR OPTIONAL FAST DAY)

Wake Up
Drink 2 large glasses of purified water with the juice of half a lemon, lime, or orange.**

Breakfast
2 sautéed (over-easy) eggs over sautéed kale, chard, spinach, collards, or dandelion greens

Dandelion root or kukicha tea

Morning Snack
Kale Muffin *(page 226)*

Dandelion root or kukicha tea

Lunch

Ultimate Green Smoothie *(page 286)*

Afternoon Snack

¹⁄₂ cup raw pumpkin seeds

Dinner

Simple Roasted Wild Salmon Fillet *(page 281)*

Roasted Cauliflower and Brussels Sprouts with Caramelized Onions and Garlic *(page 262)*

After-Dinner Snack

¹⁄₂ cup berries

Herbal tea

DAY 9

Wake Up

Drink 2 large glasses of purified water with the juice of half a lemon, lime, or orange.**

Breakfast

Ultimate Green Smoothie *(page 286)*

Morning Snack

Kale Muffin *(page 226)*

Dandelion root or kukicha tea

Lunch

Simple Curried Chickpeas and Kale *(page 267)*

Afternoon Snack

1 cup jicama slices

Dinner

Spicy Chicken with Sautéed Greens *(page 274)*

Asparagus with Dijon Sauce *(page 269)*

After-Dinner Snack

¹⁄₂ cup berries

Herbal tea

DAY 10

Wake Up
Drink 2 large glasses of purified water with the juice of half a lemon, lime, or orange.**

Breakfast
Spinach and Mushroom Omelet *(page 227)*

Dandelion root or kukicha tea

Morning Snack
Ultimate Green Smoothie *(page 286)*

Lunch
Simple Summer Salad *(page 233)*

Kale Muffin *(page 226)*

Afternoon Snack
12 almonds

Dinner
Stir-Fried Cabbage and Edamame *(page 265)*

Ginger Miso Sweet Potatoes with Sautéed Greens *(page 250)*

After-Dinner Snack
$\frac{1}{2}$ cup berries

Herbal tea

DAY 11

Wake Up
Drink 2 large glasses of purified water with the juice of half a lemon, lime, or orange.**

Breakfast
Ultimate Green Smoothie *(page 286)*

Morning Snack
Cut-up vegetables (carrots; celery; radishes; snap peas; red, yellow, orange, or green peppers) with 2 ounces hummus

Lunch
Tomato Curry Soup *(page 255)*

Adzuki Bean and Quinoa Salad with Cilantro Chile Dressing *(page 241)*

Afternoon Snack
Organic vegetable or V8 juice (can add nutritional yeast flakes* if desired)

Dinner
Grilled Thai-Style Fish *(page 282)*

Kimchi *(page 261)*

Bok Choy and Apple Salad *(page 238)*

After-Dinner Snack
½ cup berries

Herbal tea

DAY 12

Wake Up
Drink 2 large glasses of purified water with the juice of half a lemon, lime, or orange.**

Breakfast
2 or 3 soft-boiled eggs with flax seeds over greens

Dandelion root or kukicha tea

Morning Snack
1 cup jicama slices

Lunch
Yummy Black Bean Burgers *(page 244)*

Sauerkraut *(page 260)*

Crispy Roasted Kale Chips *(page 272)*

Afternoon Snack
Organic vegetable or V8 juice (can add nutritional yeast flakes* if desired)

Dinner
Chicken and Wild Mushrooms with Truffle Oil *(page 277)*

Quinoa with Lemon and Pine Nuts *(page 249)*

Kale and Brussels Sprouts Salad *(page 235)*

After-Dinner Snack
½ cup berries

Herbal tea

DAY 13

Wake Up
Drink 2 large glasses of purified water with the juice of half a lemon, lime, or orange.**

Breakfast
Ultimate Green Smoothie *(page 286)*

Morning Snack
2 hard-cooked eggs

Dandelion root or kukicha tea

Lunch
Grilled chicken

Sauerkraut *(page 260)*

Afternoon Snack
Cut-up vegetables (carrots; celery; radishes; snap peas; red, yellow, orange, or green peppers) with 2 ounces hummus

Dinner
Gazpacho *(page 254)*

Kale Muffin *(page 226)*

After-Dinner Snack
½ cup berries

Herbal tea

DAY 14

Wake Up
Drink 2 large glasses of purified water with the juice of half a lemon, lime, or orange.**

Breakfast
Spinach and Mushroom Omelet *(page 227)*

Dandelion root or kukicha tea

Morning Snack
Ultimate Green Smoothie *(page 286)*

Lunch
Tomato Curry Soup *(page 255)*

Crispy Roasted Kale Chips *(page 272)*

Afternoon Snack
¼ cup raw pumpkin seeds

Dinner
Gingered Red Snapper *(page 284)*

Roasted Brussels Sprouts with Caramelized Onions *(page 264)*

After-Dinner Snack
½ cup berries

Herbal tea

*Nutritional yeast is a complete protein that contains 18 amino acids and 15 minerals. It is a source of B vitamins that support both phases of the liver's detox process. Vitamin B_1 helps reduce the toxicity of alcohol, smoking, and heavy metals. The liver uses vitamin B_2 in the production of glutathione and B_3 in Phase One detoxification. Vitamin B_5 helps detoxify alcohol and candida overgrowth. Nutritional yeast is very helpful for vegetarians because it contains vitamin B_{12}, an essential vitamin found only in meat.

Nutritional yeast is not brewer's yeast, a by-product of the beer-making process. Nutritional yeast is grown on strains on mineral-rich molasses and absorbs the minerals from its host. Its high mineral content is healing for the liver. It is pasteurized to eliminate living yeast and will not feed candida or other yeast-related problems.

Nutritional yeast is easy to use. Just stir a tablespoon or two into vegetable or V8 juice, soups, sauces, or yogurt. It is a quick pick-me-up in the late afternoon—especially when we're forgoing that tempting venti latte or bit of dark chocolate. Stir 1 to 2 tablespoons in water for a boost of energy in 10 minutes. It has a cheesy, nutty flavor, so it's best in savory dishes rather than sweet ones.

**Water can be room temperature or hot. If possible, wait 30 to 45 minutes until breakfast.

{My LiverUp! Journal}

EAT WELL

Each day, choose one food from each of the following groups. Then use the space below to keep track of your meals.

Citrus

Lemon (½) □
Lime (½) □
Orange (1) □

Crucifers

(½ cup cooked/1 cup raw)

Broccoli □
Broccoli sprouts □
Brussels sprouts □
Cabbage □
Cauliflower □

Colon Foods (2)

Apple (1) □
Berries (1 cup) □
Carrot (1) □
Flax seed, group
(2–3 tablespoons) □
Pear (1) □
Psyllium husk
(1–2 teaspoons) □

Green Leafy

(½ cup cooked/1 cup raw)

Beet greens □
Chard □
Cilantro □
Collards □
Dandelion greens □
Escarole □
Kale □
Mustard greens □
Parsley □
Radish greens □
Watercress □

Liver Healers

Artichoke hearts (4) □
Asparagus, cooked
(½ cup) □
Beets (½ cup) □
Celery (2 ribs) □
Dandelion root tea
(1–2 cups) □
Hemp protein powder
(1–2 scoops) □
Yeast, nutritional
(1–2 teaspoons) □

Oil (1–2 tablespoons)

Coconut oil □
Flaxseed oil □
Cold-pressed olive oil □

Protein, Organic

(2 servings)

Beef □
Chicken □
Wild fish □
Lamb □
Turkey □
Veal □
Yogurt, Greek, plain □

Sulfur-Rich Foods

Daikon radish (¼ cup) □
Eggs (2) □
Garlic, 1 clove □
Onions, cooked
(½ cup) □

DRINK WATER!

My Breakfast

_____

My Lunch

_____

My Dinner

_____

My Snacks

Daily Must-Haves

Hot lemon water ☐ Dandelion tea ☐
Milk thistle supplement ☐
Water ☐☐☐☐☐☐☐☐☐☐

Move
Notes about my exercise today:

De-Stress
What steps did I take toward a calmer, more mindful life? (e.g., meditation)

Live Well
Circle the number that best matches how you feel (10 = great, 1 = poor).

Energy level	1	2	3	4	5	6	7	8	9	10
Mood	1	2	3	4	5	6	7	8	9	10
Mental focus	1	2	3	4	5	6	7	8	9	10
Sleep quality	1	2	3	4	5	6	7	8	9	10

PERSONAL NOTES

ENDNOTES

CHAPTER 2

1. Dr. John Lee, MD, *What Your Doctor May Not Tell You About: Premenopause: Balance Your Hormones and Your Life from Thirty to Fifty* (Warner Books: NY, 1999).

2. J. Fehér, A. Vereckei, G. Lengyel, "Role of free-radical reactions in liver diseases," *Acta Physiologica Hungarica.* 80, nos. 1–4 (1992): 351–61.

3. Borut Poljšak and Raja Dahmane, "Review Article: Free Radicals and Extrinsic Skin Aging," *Dermatology Research and Practice* (2012), Article ID 135206, doi. org/10.1155/2012/135206.

4. Gregory E. Miller, Sheldon Cohen, and A. Kim Ritchey, "Chronic Psychological Stress and the Regulation of Pro-Inflammatory Cytokines: A Glucocorticoid-Resistance Model," *Health Psychology* 21, No. 6.

5. Paul Pitchford, *Healing with Whole Foods: Asian Traditions and Modern Nutrition* (North Atlantic Books: Berkeley, 2002).

6. Vladimir E. Panov and Assya Krasteva, "Tongue Coating in Patients with Gastro-Intestinal and Liver Diseases," *Journal of IMAB*—Annual Proceeding (Scientific Papers) vol. 18 (2012), 2, 188–90.

7. Christopher Hobbs, *Natural Therapy for Your Liver* (Penguin Putnam: New York, 2002).

8. Pat James et al., "Understanding the Processes Behind the Regulation of Blood Glucose," *Nursing Times*, (April 2004): vol. 100, no 16: 56–58.

9. M. K. Oh, J. Winn, and F. Poordad, "Review Article: Diagnosis and Treatment of Non-alcoholic Fatty Liver Disease," *Alimentary Pharmacology and Therapetics* (January 2008) vol. 28: 503–22.

10. Saverio Stranges et al., "Body Fat Distribution, Liver Enzymes, and Risk of Hypertension Evidence From the Western New York Study," *Hypertension*, 46, no. 5 (November 2005): 1188–93.

11. G. Targher et al., "Increased Risk of CKD among Type 2 Diabetics with Nonalcoholic Fatty Liver Disease," *Journal of the American Society of Nephrology*, 2008 (19)8: 1564–70.

12. www.yalescientific.org/2011/04/research-links-sugar-consumption-fat-production -and-diabetes/

13. Leo Galland, MD, *The Fat Resistance Diet* (Broadway Books: NY, 2005).

14. Northrup, Christianne, MD, *The Wisdom of Menopause* (Bantam, NY, 2006).

15. H. B. Chae, "Alcoholic Liver Disease," *Korean Journal Gastroenterol*, May, 2009, 53 (5): 275–82.

16. William Hay, MD, *The New Health Era*, (Pacono Hay-Ven, Mt. Pocono, PA, 1933).

17. Northrup, Christianne, MD, *The Wisdom of Menopause* (Bantam, NY, 2006).

18. Amen, Daniel, MD., *Change Your Brain, Change Your Body*, (Three Rivers Press, NY, 2010).

19. Richards, Byron, CCN, *The Leptin Diet: How Fit is Your Fat?* (Truth in Wellness: Tucson, 2006).

20. Haas, Elson, *The Detox Diet* (Berkley: 10 Speed Press, 2012).

CHAPTER 3

1. Leo Galland, MD, *Power Healing* (Random House: NY, 1997).

2. M. A. Medinsky et al., "Mechanistic Considerations in Benzene Physiological Model Development," *Environ Health Perspect*. 104, suppl. 6 (December 1996): 1399–404.

3. E. M. Kenyon et al., "Differences in Rates of Benzene Metabolism Correlate with Observed Genotoxicity," *Toxicol Appl Pharmacol*. 136, no. 1 (January 1996): 49–56.

4. Sally Fallon and Mary Enig, PhD, *Nourishing Traditions* (New Trends Publishing: Washington, DC, 2001).

5. Francis Pottenger, MD, *Pottenger's Cats: A Study in Nutrition* (Price-Pottenger Nutrition Foundation: Lemon Grove, California, 1983).

6. http://www.un.org/apps/news/story.asp?NewsID=40533#.UjS-UWd2PRQ.

7. Weston Price, DDS, *Nutrition and Physical Degeneration* (Price-Pottenger Nutrition Foundation: La Mesa, California, 2000).

8. Ibid.

9. A. Furst, "Can Nutrition Affect Toxicity?" *Int J Toxicol* 21, no. 5 (September–October 2002): 419–24.

10. H. Kaya et al., "Glutathione: In Sickness and In Health," *The Lancet* 351, no. 9103 (1998): 645–46.

11. Alan Pressman, DC, PhD, CCN, *Glutathione: The Ultimate Antioxidant* (St. Martin's Press: NY, 1997).

12. D. J. Liska, PhD, and R. Rountree, MD, "The Role of Detoxification in the Prevention of Chronic Degenerative Diseases: A Summary," *Advanced Nutrition Publications*, 2002. www.livingwellsource.com/.../LWX%20OF%20dETOXIFICATION%20

13. Rogers, Sherry, MD, *Detoxify or Die* (Kensington Press: NY, 2002).

14. J. Scand, H. A. Salmi, and S. Sarna, "Effect of Silymarin on Chemical, Functional, and Morphological Alterations of the Liver. A Double-Blind Controlled Study," *Gastroenterol*. 17 no. 4 (June 1982): 517–21.

15. X. Wu, G. Beecher, J Holden, D. Haytowitz, S. Gebhardt, R. Prior, "Lipophilic and Hydrophilic Antioxidant Capacities of Common Foods in the United States," *Journal Agricultural and Food Chemistry*, 4026, no. 52 (2004) 4026–37.

CHAPTER 4

1. S. R. Knowles, E. A Nelson, and A. Palombo, "Investigating the Role of Perceived Stress on Bacterial Flora Activity and Salivary Cortisol Secretion: A Possible Mechanism Underlying Susceptibility to Illness," *Biological Psychology* 77 (2008): 132-41

2. A. Gomez et al., "Loss of Sex and Age Driven Differences in the Gut Microbiome Characterize Arthritis-Susceptible *0401 Mice but Not Arthritis-Resistant *0402 Mice," *PLoS ONE*, 7, no. 4 (2012): e36095 doi:10.1371/journal.pone.0036095.

3. http://www.npr.org/blogs/health/2013/06/18/193069110/fda-backs-off-on-regulation-of-fecal-transplants; http://www.mayoclinic.org/medicalprofs/fecal-transplants-ddue1012.html.

4. Stephanie C. Ganal et al., "Priming of Natural Killer Cells by Nonmucosal Mono-nuclear Phagocytes Requires Instructive Signals from Commensal Microbiota," *Immunity* 37, no. 1 (July 2012):171–86.

5. Natasha Campbell-McBride, MD, *Gut and Psychology Syndrome* (Medinform Publishing: UK, 2010).

6. www.dms.ufsc.br/mip7013/arquivos/25501/4Gut%20flora%20in%20health%20and%20disease.pdf.

7. K .Dylag et al., "Probiotics in the Mechanism of Protection against Gut Inflamma-tion and Therapy of Gastrointestinal Disorders," *Curr Pharm Des.* (Jun 10, 2013).

8. Paul Pitchford, *Healing with Whole Foods* (North Atlantic Books: Berkeley, 2002).

9. Ibid.

10. Andres Gomez, et al., "Loss of Sex and Age Driven Differences in the Gut Microbi-ome Characterize Arthritis-Susceptible *0401 Mice but Not Arthritis-Resistant *0402 Mice," *PLoS ONE* 7, no. 4 (2012): e36095, doi:10.1371/journal.pone.0036095

11. http://www.scientificamerican.com/article.cfm?id=strange-but-true-humans-carry-more-bacterial-cells-than-human-ones&page=2.

12. Francisco Guarner and Juan-R Malagelada, "Gut Flora in Health and Disease," *The Lancet* 361, no. 9356 (February 8, 2003): 512–19.

13. Paul Pitchford, *Healing with Whole Foods* (North Atlantic Books: Berkeley, 2002).

14. Guarner, "Gut Flora in Health and Disease."

15. J. B. Furness, W. A. Kunze, and N. Clerc, "Nutrient Tasting and Signaling Mecha-nisms in the Gut. II. The Intestine as a Sensory Organ: Neural, Endocrine, and Immune Responses," *Am J Physiol.* 277, no .5, pt. 1 (November 1999): G922–28.

16. http://mayoresearch.mayo.edu/center-for-individualized-medicine/microbiome-program.asp

17. Scott H Podolsky, "Metchnikoff and the Microbiome, "*The Lancet* 380, iss. 9856 (November 24, 2012): 1810–11, doi:10.1016/S0140-6736(12)62018-22.

18. http://www.scientificamerican.com/article/strange-but-true-humans-carry-more-bacterial-cells-than-human-ones/

19. K . Dylag, M. Hubalewska-Mazgaj, M. Surmiak, J. Szmyd, and T Brzozowski, "Probiotics in the Mechanism of Protection against Gut inflammation and Therapy of Gastrointestinal Disorders," *Curr Pharm Des.*, published electronically June 10, 2013.

20. Ibid.

21. D. Wagner and S Johnson, "Probiotic *lactobacillus* and estrogen effects on vaginal epithelial gene expression responses to Candida albicans," *Journal of Biomedical Science*, 2012, 19 (58).

22. A. J. Cox , D. B. Pyne , P. U. Saunders, P. A. Fricker, "Oral administration of the probiotic Lactobacillus fermentum VRI-003 and mucosal immunity in endurance athletes,"*British Journal Sports Medicine*, 2010 Mar; 44 (4): 222–26.

23. S. S. Biradar, S. T. Bahagvati, and B. Shegunshi, "Probiotics and Antibiotics: A Brief Overview," *Internet Journal of Nutrition and Wellness* 2, no. 1 (2005): doi:10.5580/fc0.

24. C. M. Whisner et al., "Galacto-oligosaccharides Increase Calcium Absorption and Gut Bifidobacteria in Young Girls: A Double-Blind Cross-Over Trial, *Br J Nutr.* 110, no. 7 (October 2013): 1292–303, doi:10.1017/S000711451300055X.

25. G. R. Gibson and M. B. Roberfroid, "Dietary Modulation of the Human Colonic Microbiota: Introducing the Concept of Prebiotics," *Journal of Nutrition* 125, no. 6 (July 1995): 1401–12.

26. Carlo Selmi et al., "The Effects of Spirulina on Anemia and Immune Function in Senior Citizens," *Cellular & Molecular Immunology* 8 (May 2011): 248–254, doi:10.1038/cmi.2010.76.

27. Eun Hee Lee, Ji-Eun Park, Young-Ju Choi, Kap-Bum Huh, and Wha-Young Kim, "A Randomized Study to Establish the Effects of Spirulina in Type 2 Diabetes Mellitus Patients," *Nutr Res Pract.* 2, no. 4 (Winter 2008): 295–300.

28. Randall E. Merchant, Charles D. Rice, and Harold F. Young, "Dietary Chlorella Pyrenoidosa for Patients with Malignant Glioma: Effects on Immunocompetence, Quality of Life, and Survival," *Phytotherapy Research* 4, iss. 6 (December 1990): 220–31.

29. Paul Pitchford, *Healing with Whole Foods* (North Atlantic Books: Berkeley, 2002).

30. *The Yoga Sutras of Patanjali*, Translation and Commentary by Sri Swami Satchidananda (Integral Yoga Publications, Yogaville, VA, 1999).

CHAPTER 5

1. http://lpi.oregonstate.edu/f-w00/flavonoid.html.

2. John D. Clarke, Anna Hsu, Zhen Yu, Roderick H. Dashwood, and Emily Ho, "Differential Effects of Sulforaphane on Histone Deacetylases, Cell Cycle Arrest and Apoptosis in Normal Prostate Cells versus Hyperplastic and Cancerous Prostate Cells," *Molecular Nutrition and Food Research*, 55(7): 999–1009 (2011); doi:10.1002/mnfr.201000547.

3. E. G. Rogan, "The Natural Chemopreventive Compound Indole-3-Carbinol: State of the Science," *In Vivo* 20, no. 2 (March–April 2006): 221–28.

4. J. H. Fowke, J. D. Morrow, S. Motley, R. M. Bostick, and R. M. Ness, "Brassica Vegetable Consumption Reduces Urinary F2-Isoprostane Levels Independent of Micronutrient Intake," *Carcinogenesis* 27, no. 10 (October 2006): 2096–102, published electronically May 15, 2006.

5. Mark Stengler, ND, *The Natural Physician's Healing Therapies* (Prentice-Hall Press: NY, 2001).

6. Paul Pitchford, *Healing with Whole Foods* (North Atlantic Books: Berkeley, 2002).

7. Tanaka et al., "Studies on Inhibition of Intestinal Absorption of Radio-Active Strontium," *Canadian Medical Association Journal* 99:169-75, 1968.

8. Pitchford, *Healing with Whole Foods*.

9. J. K. Chavan and S. S. Kadan, "Nutritional Improvement of Cereals by Sprouting," *Critical Reviews in Food Science and Nutrition* 28, no. 5 (1989): 401–37.

10. Ibid.

11. D. J. Peer and S. Leeson, "Feeding Value of Hydroponically Sprouted Barley for Poultry and Pigs," *Animal Feed Science and Technology* 13, no. 3–4 (December 1985): 183–190.

12. Chavan, "Nutritional Improvement of Cereals by Sprouting."

13. J. W. Fah, Y. Zhang, and P. Talaley, "Broccoli Sprouts: An Exceptionally Rich Source of Inducers of Enzymes that Protect against Chemical Carcinogens," *Proc. Natl. Acad. Sci. USA*, 94 (September 1997): 10367–72.

14. I. F. Robey et al., "Bicarbonate Increases Tumor pH and Inhibits Spontaneous Metastases," Cancer Res. 69, no. 6 (March 15, 2009): 2260–68, doi:10.1158/0008-5472.CAN-07-5575.

15. W. Qidwai and T. Ashfaq, "Role of Garlic Usage in Cardiovascular Disease Prevention: An Evidence-Based Approach," *Evidence-Based Complementary and Alternative Medicine*, 2013 (March 2013), Article ID 125649.

16. A. J. Manonmani, A. Abraham, and M. P. Narmadha, "Effect of Silymarin in Diabetes Mellitus Patients with Liver Diseases, *Journal of Pharmacology and Pharmacotherapeutics*.

17. R. Gebhardt, "Inhibition of Cholesterol Biosynthesis in Primary Cultured Rat Hepatocytes by Artichoke (*Cynara scolymus* L.) Extracts," *J Pharmacol Exp Ther* 286 (1999):1122–28.

18. A. T. Borchers, J. S. Stern, R. M. Hackman, C. L. Keen, and M. E. Gershwin, "Mushrooms, Tumors, and Immunity," *Proc Soc Exp Biol Med.* 221, no. 4 (September, 1999): 281–93.

19. Okezie I. Aruoma, L. Stephen Coles, Bernie Landes, and John E. Repine, "Characteristics and Bioefficacy of Ergothioneine—A Unique Natural Dietary Antioxidant," *e-Journal of Age Management Medicine*; 6, no. 5 (May 2011): http://www.agemed.org/AMMGejournal/May2011.aspx.

20. C. Gemma, J. Vila, A. Bachstetter, and P. Bickford, *Brain Aging: Models, Methods, and Mechanisms* (CRC Press: Boca Raton, 2007), chapter 15.

21. J. Joseph et al., "Reversals of Age-Related Declines in Neuronal Signal Transduction, Cognitive, and Motor Behavioral Deficits with Blueberry, Spinach, or Strawberry Dietary Supplementation," *Journal of Neuroscience* 19, no. 18 (Sept.,1999): 8114–21.

22. Aedin Cassidy et al., "High Anthocyanin Intake Is Associated with a Reduced Risk of Myocardial Infarction in Young and Middle-Aged Women," *Circulation: Journal of the American Heart Association* 127 (February 2013): 188–96.

23. A. Bishayee A et al., "Anthocyanin-Rich Black Currant Extract Suppresses the Growth of Human Hepatocellular Carcinoma Cells," *Nat Prod Commun* 5, no. 10 (October 2010): 1613–18.

24. Ibid.

25. http://www.health.mil/dhb/downloads/2011/Hibbeln1/4Defence%20Health%20Board%20NOV%2014%20%202011%20as%20presented.pdf.

26. http://www.coconutresearchcenter.org/article10612.htm.

27. Mary Enig, PhD, and Sally Fallon, Sally, *Eat Fat Lose Fat* (Hudson Street Press: New York, 2005).

28. Z. Li et al., "Hass Avocado Modulates Postprandial Vascular Reactivity and Post-prandial Inflammatory Responses to a Hamburger Meal in Healthy Volunteers," *Food Funct.* 4, no. 3 (February 26, 2013): 384–91, doi:10.1039/c2fo30226h.

29. Maria-Isabel Covas et al., "The Effect of Polyphenols in Olive Oil on Heart Disease Risk Factors: A Randomized Trial," *Annals of Internal Medicine* 145, no. 5 (September 5, 2006): 333–41.

30. B. Furhman et al., "Ginger Extract Consumption Reduces Plasma Cholesterol, Inhibits LDL Oxidation, and Attenuates Development of Atherrosclorosis in Atherosclerotic, Apolipoprotein E-deficient mice," *Journal of Nutrition* 130 (2000): 1124–31.

31. A. Kode, R. Rajagopalan, S. V. Penumathsa, and V. P. Menon, "Effect of Ethanol and Thermally Oxidized Sunflower Oil Ingestion on Phospholipid Fatty Acid Composition of Rat Liver: Protective Role of Cuminum cyminum L.," *Ann Nutr Metab.* 49, no. 5 (September-October 2005): 300–303.

32. S. Satyanarayana, K. Sushruta, G. S. Sarma, N. Srinivas, and G. V. Subba Raju, "Antioxidant Activity of the Aqueous Extracts of Spicy Food Additives—Evaluation and Comparison with Ascorbic Acid in In-Vitro Systems," *J Herb Pharmacother* 4, no. 2 (2004): 1–10.

33. P. Dhanapakiam, J. M. Joseph, V. K. Ramaswamy, M. Moorthi, and A. S. Kumar, "The Cholesterol Lowering Property of Coriander Seeds (*Coriandrum sativum*): Mechanism of Action," *J Environ Biol.* 29, no. 1 (January 2008): 53–56.

34. http://customers.hbci.com/~wenonah/new/9steps.htm.

35. Anna Baghdasaryan et al., "Curcumin Improves Sclerosing Cholangitis in Mdr2-/- Mice by Inhibition of Cholangiocyte Inflammatory Response and Portal Myofibroblast Proliferation," *Gut* 59 (2010): 521–530, doi:10.1136/gut.2009.186528.

36. Nora Gedgaudas, CNS, CNT, *Primal Body, Primal Mind* (Healing Arts Press: Rochester, VT, 2011).

37. Mark Bittman, *Food Matters: A Guide to Conscious Eating* (Simon and Schuster: NY, 2009).

38. http://www.ams.usda.gov/AMSv1.0/ams.fetchTemplateData.do?template=TemplateC &leftNav=NationalOrganicProgram&page=NOPConsumers&description=Consumers

39. http://www.ucsusa.org/food1/4and1/4agriculture/solutions/advance-sustainable -agriculture/greener-pastures.html

40. http://www.mayoclinic.com/health/grass-fed-beef/AN02053

41. Paul Pitchford, *Healing with Whole Foods* (North Atlantic Books: Berkley, 2002).

42. W. F. Lai, "Nucleic Acid Therapy for Lifespan Prolongation: Present and Future," *J Biosci.* 36, no. 4 (September 2011): 725–29.

43. Pitchford, *Healing with Whole Foods.*

44. Ibid.

45. F. B. Hu and M. J. Stampher, "Nut Consumption and Risk of Coronary Heart Disease: A Review of Epicemiologic Evidence," *Current Atherosclerosis Reports*, 1, no. 3 (November 1999): 204–9.

46. Kathleen DesMaisons, PhD, *Potatoes Not Prozac* (Simon and Schuster: NY, 2008).

47. http://www.umm.edu/altmed/articles/milk-thistle-000266.htm

48. Ibid.

49. Ibid.

50. Michael Moss, *Salt Sugar Fat: How the Food Giants Hooked Us,* (Random House: NY, 2013).

51. Kimber L. Stanhope, et al., "Consumption of Fructose and High Fructose Corn Syrup Increase Postprandial Triglycerides, LDL-Cholesterol, and Apolipoprotein-B in Young Men and Women," *Journal of Clinical Endocrinal Metabolism* 96, no. 10 (October 2011): E1596–E1605.

52. Kiyah J. Duffey and Barry M. Popkin, "High-Fructose Corn Syrup: Is This What's for Dinner?" *Am J Clin Nutr.* 88, no. 6 (December 2008): 1722S–1732S, doi:10.3945/ajcn.2008.25825C PMCID: PMC2746720NIHMSID: NIHMS98834.

53. www.cdc.gov/obesity/downloads/obesity1/4trends1/42010.pdf

54. William Davis, MD, *Wheat Belly* (Rodale: Emmaus, PA, 2011).

55. Ibid.

56. Enig, *Eat Fat Lose Fat.*

57. http://envirocancer.cornell.edu/factsheet/diet/fs1.phyto.cfm.

58. Ibid.

59. V. Chatsudthipong and C. Muanprasat, "Stevioside and related compounds: therapeutic benefits beyond sweetness," *Pharmacol Ther.* 121, no. 1 (January 2009): 41–54, doi:10.1016/j.pharmthera.2008.09.007.

CHAPTER 6

1. Paramahansa Yogananda, *Man's Eternal Quest: Collected Talks and Essays on Realizing God in Daily Life, Volume I* (Self Realization Fellowship: Los Angeles, 2001).

2. Edmond Bordeaux Szekely, editor and translator, *The Essene Gospel of Peace* (Academy of Creative Living: Denver, 1971).

3. Alexis M. Stranahan and Mark P. Mattson, "Recruiting Adaptive Cellular Stress Responses for Successful Brain Ageing," *Nature Reviews Neuroscience* 13 (March 2012): 209–16.

4. http://hub.jhu.edu/magazine/2012/summer/dont-feed-your-head.

5. Dr. Michael Mosley and Mimi Spencer, *The Fast Diet* (Atria Books: New York, 2013).

6. Monica C. Klempel, Cynthia M. Kroeger, and Krista A. Varady, "Alternate Day Fasting (ADF) with a High-Fat Diet Produces Similar Weight Loss and Cardio-Protection as ADF with a Low-Fat Diet," *Metabolism—Clinical and Experimental* 62, no. 1 (January 2013): 137–43.

7. Megumi Hatori et al., "Time-Restricted Feeding without Reducing Caloric Intake Prevents Metabolic Diseases in Mice Fed a High-Fat Diet," *Cell Metabolism*, 15, no. 6 (May 17, 2012): 848–60.

8. Ibid.

9. Ibid.

10. Ibid.

11. Di Ma, Satchidananda Panda, and Jiandie D Lin, "Temporal Orchestration of Circadian Autophagy Rhythm by C/EBPß," *EMBO Journal* 30, no. 22 (November 16, 2011): 4642–51.

12. Bérengère Coupé et al., "Loss of Autophagy in Pro-opiomelanocortin Neurons Perturbs Axon Growth and Causes Metabolic Dysregulation," *Cell Metabolism* 15, no. 2, (January 26, 2012): 247–55.

13. Ibid.

14. Joel Fuhrman, MD, *Fasting and Eating for Health* (St. Martin's Press: New York, 1995).

15. Martin Bronwen, Mark P. Mattson, and Stuart Maudsley, "Caloric Restriction and Intermittent Fasting: Two Potential Diets for Successful Brain Aging," *Ageing Res Rev.* 5, no. 3 (August 2006): 332–53.

16. Ibid.

17. Russell Jaffe, MD, PhD, "The Alkaline Way in Digestive Health," in *Bioactive Food as Dietary Interventions for Liver and Gastrointestinal Disease*, edited by Ronald Ross Watson and Victor R. Preedy (San Diego: Academic Press, 2013), 1–2.

18. Martin Bronwen, Mark P. Mattson, and Stuart Maudsley, "Caloric Restriction and Intermittent Fasting: Two Potential Diets for Successful Brain Aging," *Ageing Res Rev.* 5, no. 3 (August 2006): 332–53.

19. Elson Haas, MD, *Staying Healthy with Nutrition* (Crown Publishing: New York, 2006), 740.

20. Ibid, 70.

21. http://www.treeoflife.nu/DRCOUSENS/DRCOUSENSBLOG/tabid/364 /language/en-US/~/Default.aspx?tabid=364&PostID=167&language=en-US

22. S. M. Ghosh et al., "Enhanced Vasodilator Activity of Nitrite in Hypertension—Critical Role for Erythrocytic Xanthine Oxidoreductase and Translational Potential," *Hypertension* 61 (2013): 1091–1102; doi:10.1161/HYPERTENSIONAHA.111.00933.

23. Q. Dai, A. R. Borenstein, Y. Wu, J. C. Jackson, and E. B. Larson, "Fruit and Vegetable Juices and Alzheimer's Disease: The Kame Project," *Am J Med.* 119, no. 9 (September 2006): 751–59.

24. Stanley Burroughs, *The Master Cleanser* (SnowballPublishing.com, 2013).

25. J. E. Galgani and E. Ravussin, "Effect of Dihydrocapsiate on Resting Metabolic Rate in Humans," *Am J Clin Nutr.* 92, no. 5 (November 2010): 1089–93.

26. S. Whiting, E. Derbyshire, B. K. Tiwari, "Capsaicinoids and Capsinoids. A Potential Role for Weight Management? A Systematic Review of the Evidence," *Journal Appetite* 59, no. 2 (October 2012): 341–48; T. Yoneshiro, S. Aita, Y. Kawai, T. Iwanaga, and M. Saito, "Nonpungent Capsaicin Analogs (Capsinoids) Increase Energy Expenditure through the Activation of Brown Adipose Tissue in Humans." *American Journal Clinical Nutrition*, 95, no. 4 (April 2012): 845–50; H.C. Reinbach, A. Smeets, T. Martinussen, P. Møller, and M.S. Westerterp-Plantenga, "Effects of Capsaicin, Green Tea and CH-19 Sweet Pepper on Appetite and Energy Intake in Humans in Negative and Positive Energy Balance," *Journal of Clinical Nutrition* 28 (2009): 260–65.

27. S. Maggini, S. Beveridge, M. Suter, "A Combination of High-Dose Vitamin C plus Zinc for the Common Cold," *J Int Med Res.* 40, no. 1 (2012): 28–42; *Mini Rev Med Chem.* 2012 Jan;12(1):35-43. Ascorbic acid: an old player with a broad impact on body physiology including oxidative stress suppression and immunomodulation: a review. Pohanka M, Pejchal J, Snopkova S, Havlickova K, Karasova JZ, Bostik P, Pikula J.; D.E. Okwu and I.N. Emenike, "Evaluation of the Phytonutrients and Vitamin Content of Citrus Fruits," *International Journal of Molecular Medicine and Advanced Sciences* 2, no. 1 (2006): 1–6; John L. Beard, "Iron Biology in Immune Function, Muscle Metabolism and Neuronal Functioning," *J. Nutr.* 131, no. 2 (February 1, 2001): 568S–580S.

28. M. I. Gil, F. A. Tomas-Barberan, B. Hess-Pierce, D. M. Holcroft, and A. A. Kader, "Antioxidant Activity of Pomegranate Juice and Its Relationship with Phenolic Composition and Processing," *J Agric Food Chem.* 48, no. 10 (2000): 4581–89.

29. M. Aviram et al., "Pomegranate Juice Consumption for 3 years by Patients with Carotid Artery Stenosis Reduces Common Carotid Intima-Media Thickness, Blood Pressure and LDL oxidation," *Clinical Nutrition* 23, no. 3 (June 2004):423–33.

30. Mira Rosenblat, Nina Volkova, and Michael Aviram, "Pomegranate Phytosterol (ß-sitosterol) and Polyphenolic Antioxidant (Punicalagin) Addition to Statin, Significantly Protected against Macrophage Foam Cells Formation," *Atherosclerosis* 226, no. 1 (January 2013): 110–11.

31. Yiming Li et al., "Preventive and Protective Properties of Zingiber officinale (Ginger) in Diabetes Mellitus, Diabetic Complications, and Associated Lipid and Other Metabolic Disorders: A Brief Review, Evid Based Complement," *Alternat Med.* 2012:516870.

32. Amirhossein Sahebkar, "Potential Efficacy of Ginger as a Natural Supplement for Nonalcoholic Fatty Liver Disease," *World J Gastroenterol.* 17, no. 2 (January 14, 2011): 271–72.

33. A. H. Atta et al., "Hepatoprotective Effect of Methanol Extracts of Zingiber officinale and Cichorium intybus," *Indian Journal of Pharmaceutical Science* 72, no. 5 (September–October 2010): 564–70.

34. Ghada M. Nobil, Atef M.M. Attia, and M.A. Elhag, "Radioprotective Effects of Dietary Ginger (Zingiber officinale) Against Fast Neutron-Induced Oxidative Stress in Rats," *World Applied Sciences Journal* 6, no. 4 (2009): 494–98.

35. Ashley Magistrelli and Jo Carol Chezem, "Effect of Ground Cinnamon on Postprandial Blood Glucose Concentration in Normal-Weight and Obese Adults," *RD J Acad Nutr Diet.* 112 (2012): 1806–9; A. C. Skulas-Ray, P. M. Kris-Etherton, D. L. Teeter, et al. "A High Antioxidant Spice Blend Attenuates Postprandial Insulin and Triglyceride Responses and Increases Some Plasma Measures of Antioxidant Activity in Healthy, Overweight Men," *J Nutr* 141, no. 8 (August 2011): 1451–57.

36. http://lpi.oregonstate.edu/infocenter/minerals/manganese/

37. K. E. Tanguay, S. T. Mortimer, P. H. Wood, and D. A. Hanley, "The Effects of Phorbol Myristate Acetate on the Intracellular Degradation of Bovine Parathyroid Hormone," *Endocrinology* 128, no. 4 (April 1991): 1863–68.

38. D. L. Baly, J. S. Schneiderman, and A. L. Garcia-Welsh, "Effect of Manganese Deficiency on Insulin Binding, Glucose Transport and Metabolism in Rat Adipocytes," *Journal of Nutrition* 120, no. 9 (1990): 1075–79.

39. Norlaily Mohd Ali et al., "The Promising Future of Chia, Salvia hispanica L.," *Journal of Biomedical Biotechnology* (2012): 171956.

40. Jocelynn E. Thomas and Michael J. Glade, "Stevia: It's Not Just About Calories," *Open Obesity Journal* 2 (2010): 101–9.

CHAPTER 7

1. Gabriel Cousens, MD, *Spiritual Nutrition* (North Atlantic Books: Berkley, 2005), 341–42.

2. Dalai Lama and Howard Cutler, MD, *Art of Happiness* (The Penguin Group: New York, 1998), 41.

3. Micheal Gershon, MD, *The Second Brain* (Harper Collins: New York, 1998).

4. Ibid.

5. http://www.nytimes.com/2005/08/23/health/23gut.html?pagewanted=all&1/4r=0

6. Ibid.

7. Ibid.

8. Jon Kabat-Zinn, *Coming to Our Senses* (The Penguin Group: New York, 2007).

9. Jon Kabat-Zinn, *Wherever You Go, There You Are* (Hyperion: New York, 2009), 53.

10. Fernando Gómez-Pinilla, "Science and Society: Brain Foods: The Effects of Nutrients on Brain Function," *Nature Reviews Neuroscience* 9 (July 2008): 568–78.

11. Thich Nhat Hanh, *Peace Is Every Breath* (Harper Collins: New York, 2011), 5.

12. Ibid.

13. http://www.mayoclinic.com/health/food-and-mood/my00716.

14. Jeffery A. Dusek and Herbert Benson, "Mind-Body Medicine A Model of the Comparative Clinical Impact of the Acute Stress and Relaxation Responses," *Minn Med.* 92, no. 5 (May 2009): 47–50.

15. Mark Liponis, MD, *UltraLongevity* (Little Brown: New York, 2007).

16. http://www.psychologytoday.com/blog/the-athletes-way/201302/the-neurobiology-grace-under-pressure.

17. V. A. Pavlov and K. J. Tracey, "The Cholinergic Anti-Inflammatory Pathway," *Brain Behav Immun.* 19, no. 6 (November 2005): 493–99.

18. N. D. Theise and R. Harris, "Postmodern Biology: (Adult) (Stem) Cells are Plastic, Stochastic, Complex, and Uncertain," *Handb Exp Pharmacol* 175 (2006): 389–408.

19. Britta K. Hölzel et al., "Mindfulness Practice Leads to Increases in Regional Brain Gray Matter Density," *Psychiatry Research: Neuroimaging* 191, no. 1 (2011): 36–43.

20. Ibid.

21. Erica M.S. Sibinga, "Mindfulness-Based Stress Reduction for Urban Youth," *J Altern Complement Med.* 17, no. 3 (March 2011): 213–18.

22. Thich Nhat Hanh, *Peace Is Every Step.* (Harper Collins: New York, 2011). p. 11.

23. R. Jerath, J. W. Edry, V. A. Barnes, and V. Jerath, "Physiology of Long Pranayamic Breathing: Neural Respiratory Elements May Provide a Mechanism That Explains How Slow Deep Breathing Shifts the Autonomic Nervous System," *Med Hypotheses* 67, no. 3 (2006): 566-71, published electronically April 18, 2006.

24. E. H. Ricanati et al., "Mitigating Preventable Chronic Disease: Progress Report of the Cleveland Clinic's Lifestyle 180 Program," *Nutr Metab (Lond).* 8 (November 23, 2011): 83, doi:10.1186/1743-7075-8-83.

25. H. A. Slagter, R. J. Davidson, et al., "Mental Training Affects Distribution of Limited Brain Resources," *PLoS Biol* 5, no. 6 (2007): e138, doi:10.1371/journal.pbio.0050138.

26. D. E. Anderson, J. D. McNeely, M. A. Chesney, and B. G. Windham, "Breathing Variability at Rest is Positively Associated with 24-h Blood Pressure Level," *Am J Hypertens.* 21, no. 12 (December 2008): 1324–29, doi:10.1038/ajh.2008.292.

27. Ibid.

28. Ibid.

29. Beck Charlotte Joko, *Everyday Zen* (Harper Collins: San Francisco, 1989).

30. Kornfield, Jack, *A Path with Heart: A Guide Through the Perils and Promises of Spiritual Life* (Bantam: NY, 1993).

31. Annie Lamott, *Traveling Mercies* (Random House: New York, 1999).

32. Ehren R. Dodson and Phyllis C. Zee, "Therapeutics for Circadian Rhythm Sleep Disorders," *Sleep Med Clin.* 5, no. 4 (December 2010): 701–15.

33. http://www.epsomsaltcouncil.org/articles/report1/4on1/4absorption1/4of1/4magnesium1/4sulfate.pdf.

34. S. J. Genuis, D. Birkholz, I. Rodushkin, S. Beesoon, "Blood, urine, and sweat (BUS) Study: Monitoring and Elimination of Bioaccumulated Toxic Elements," *Archives of Environmental Contamination and Toxicology.* 2011 Aug; 61 (2): 344–57.

35. M. Toda, R. Den, M. Hasegawa-Ohira, and K. Morimoto, "Effects of Woodland Walking on Salivary Stress Markers Cortisol and Chromogranin," *Complementary Therapies in Medicine* 21, no. 1 (February 2013): 29–34.

36. K. A. Reich, Y. W. Chen, P. D. Thompson, E. P. Hoffman, P. M. Clarkson, "Forty-Eight Hours of Unloading and 24 h of Reloading Lead to Changes in Global Gene

Expression Patterns Related to Ubiquitination and Oxidative Stress in Humans," *J Appl Physiol*. 109, no. 5 (November 2010): 1404–15, doi:10.1152/japplphysiol.00444.2010.

37. D. W. Dunstan et al., "Breaking Up Prolonged Sitting Reduces Postprandial Glucose and Insulin Responses," *Diabetes Care* 35, no. 5 (May 2012): 976–83, doi:10.2337/dc11-1931.

38. Michael Pollan, *Cooked: A Natural History of Transformation* (Penguin Press: New York, 2013).

CHAPTER 8

1. B. K. S. Iyengar, *Light on Yoga* (Schocken Books: New York, 1979).

2. S. B. Khalsa, S. M. Shorter, S. Cope, G. Wyshak, and E. Sklar, "Yoga Ameliorates Performance Anxiety and Mood Disturbance in Young Professional Musicians," *Appl Psychophysiol Biofeedback* 34, no. 4 (December 2009): 279–89, doi:10.1007/s10484-009-9103-4.

3. http://www.forbes.com/sites/alicegwalton/2011/06/16/penetrating-postures-the-science-of-yoga/.

4. M. Balasubramaniam, S. Telles. and P. Murali Doraiswamy, "Yoga on Our Minds: A Systematic Review of Yoga for Neuropsychiatric Disorders," *Front. Psychiatry* 3 (January 25, 2013): 117, doi:10.3389/fpsyt.2012.00117.

CHAPTER 10

1. http://www.prevention.com/food/healthy-eating-tips/12-commonly-contaminated-foods

INDEX

Underscored page references indicate boxed text. **Boldface** references indicate illustrations.

Hydrogenated oils, 126
Hypertension, 36, 147–48, 156–57, 171

I

Immune system
  autoimmune responses, 26–27, 75, 78
  function of, 7–8, 10, 28, 85
  gut flora and, 77
Indigestion, 29–31
Indoles, 95
Inflammation, 7–8, 10, 26–29, 75, 106, 195
Inflammatory bowel disease, 75
Inflammatory cascade, 27–28
Inhibitory breathing, 181
Insulin levels, 32, 33–34, 125, 171–72
Intentionality, 170. *See also* Mindfulness
Intestinal nervous system, 164–65, 168–69
Inulin, 104, 122

J

Jaundice, 42
Jerusalem artichokes, 104
Joint pain, 19, 27–29
Journaling, 92, 170, 295, 299, 312–13
Juicing. *See also* Fasting
  recipes, 150–51, 153
  tips for, 148

K

Kale
  health benefits, 97
  recipes using
    Apple Power juice, 151
    Crispy Roasted Kale Chips, 272
    Ginger Smoothie, 291
    Green Pom Cooler juice, 151
    Green Pom Seed juice, 151
    Hearty Cleansing Soup, 251
    Kale, Squash, and White Bean Salad, 243
    Kale and Brussels Sprouts Salad, 235
    Kale Slaw with Red Cabbage and Carrots,
      266
    Nannie's Healing Chicken Soup, 259
    Power Smoothie, 287
    Purple Power Smoothie, 289
    Sassy Smoothie, 292
    Simple Curried Chickpeas and Kale, 267
    Spicy Kale juice, 150

Kefir, 86
Kidney function, 30, 36–37
Kimchi
  health benefits, 86, 104
  recipe for, 261
Kombucha tea, 86

L

Labeling issues, 114
Lactase, 125
Lactobacteria, 76
Lauric acid, 107
LDL, 37–38, 100, 101, 110
Leaky gut syndrome, 77–78
Lecithin, 101
Leeks, 100
Legumes, sprouting of, 67
Lemons
  Apple Power juice, 151
  Asparagus with Toasted Pine Nuts and
    Lemon Peel, 268
  health benefits, 89, 154
  in juicing, 151
  Master Cleanse Lemonade, 153
  Quinoa with Lemon and Pine Nuts, 249
Lentil Salad, 230
L-ergothioneine, 102
Lipid-soluble chemicals, 6, 39, 47–48, 298
Liver
  anatomy, 3–4, **4**
  disease of/damage to, 21, 157
  fasting and, 141–42
  function of
    filtering mechanisms, 3–10, 26–27
    hormone regulation, 16–17, 39–40
    nutrient processing, 10–16
    overview, 1–3, 18
  health quiz, 22–23
  sluggish/toxic, symptoms, 22–24
Liver enzymes, 21
LiverUp! Cleanse
  benefits, 44, 86–87
  follow-up, 296–99
  food groups in, 90–91, 115, 120–22
  foods to avoid, 91, 123–130
  gut-healing principles, 80–86
  mindfulness and, 163–64
  optional fast, 146–160
  overview, 89, 92, 130–31
  self-evaluation, 295–96

Sulfhydryl, 57
Sulforaphane, 95, 98
Sulfur, 57, 96, 100–102, 142
Sulfur-based amino acids, _59_
Sunchokes, 104
Sunflower seeds, _118_
Superoxide dismutase, 56–57, 158
Supplements, fasting and, _158_
Sweeteners, 31, 122, 123–25, _124_, 130
Sweet potatoes
    Ginger Miso Sweet Potatoes with Sautéed
        Greens, 250
    in LiverUp! Cleanse, _91_, 121–22
    One-Pot Chicken with Garlic and Winter
        Vegetables, 279
Swelling, of tissues, 27
Synapse function, 166–67

T

Taraxacin, 97
Taurine, _59_
Tea, 86, 122, 190
Tempeh, 85–86, _118_
Tomatoes
    Gazpacho, 254
    Hearty Cleansing Soup, 251
    Tomato Curry Soup, 255
Tongue, coated, 29
Toxins
    removal of, 14 (_see also_ Detoxification)
    sources of, 5–7, _8_, _9_, _48_, _124_
Trans fats, 125–26, 166–67
Triglycerides, _32_, 38, 107, 123–24
Tryptophan, 168–69
Turmeric, _65_, 111. _See also_ Curcumin
12-Day LiverUp! Cleanse. _See_ LiverUp!
    Cleanse
Tylenol, 41–42
Type 2 diabetes, 36–37, 84, 125

U

Ulmer, Tracy, **293**, _293_
Urea, 7, 30

V

Vagus nerve, 172
Vegan diets, _55_, _59_

Vegetable oils, 60
Vegetables. _See also_ Vegetable side dishes
    cruciferous, _54_, _58_, _90_, 94–96, 104–5
    cultured foods, 104–5
    health benefits, _54_, _58_, _90_, _298–99_
    juicing of, 148–49, _150–51_ (_see also_
        Smoothie recipes)
    leafy dark greens, _90_, 96–97
    organic, _94_, _148_
    as protein source, 119–120
    sea vegetables, _90_, 97–98
Vegetable side dishes. _See also_ Salad recipes
    Asparagus with Dijon Sauce, 269
    Asparagus with Toasted Pine Nuts and
        Lemon Peel, 268
    Crispy Roasted Kale Chips, 272
    Kimchi, 261
    One-Pot Chicken with Garlic and Winter
        Vegetables, 279
    Roasted Asparagus, 271
    Roasted Brussels Sprouts with Caramelized
        Onions, 264
    Roasted Cauliflower, Broccolini, and
        Chickpeas, 263
    Roasted Cauliflower and Brussels Sprouts
        with Caramelized Onions and Garlic,
        262
    Sauerkraut, 260
    Simple Curried Chickpeas and Kale,
        267
    Stir-Fried Cabbage and Edamame, 265
Vegetarian diets, _55_, _59_, 85–86, _311_
Victor, Martha, **300**, _300_
Vitamin A, 63, 95
Vitamin B complex, 85, 98
Vitamin C, _54_, 63, 89, 128, 154
Vitamin E, 63
Vitamin K, 96
Vitamins, fat-soluble, 15, 30–31

W

Walnuts, 121
Water consumption, _90_, 92–94, _93_
Watercress
    Freshener juice, _150_
    Watercress Salad, 231
    Watercress Soup, 252
Water-soluble chemicals, 6, 48, 60
"Weeding," in gut healing, 80